Hold on tight to your rope,
don't lose hope;
it truly is possible to recover your children.

A Ship in the Storm
The Puzzle of Autism

Disclaimer: This information is presented by independent medical experts whose sources of information include studies from the world's medical and scientific literature, patient records, and other clinical and anecdotal reports. All dosages listed are based on the authors' personal experiences. It is important to note that each person's body type and tolerance levels to supplements may be somewhat different. The publisher, authors, and/or experts specifically cited in this publication are not responsible for any consequences, direct or indirect, resulting from any reader's action(s). This book is not intended to be a substitute for consultation with a health care provider. You, the reader are instructed to consult with your personal health care provider prior to acting on any suggestions contained in this book. The purpose of this publication is to educate the reader. The material in this book is for informational purposes only and is not intended for the diagnosis or treatment of disease.

Reprint – 3rd Edition

ISBN: 0-9759674-4-4
Matrix Development Publishing
Payson, Arizona

The Puzzle of Autism:

Putting It All Together

A Guide to Transforming the

Treatment of Autism

For Parents and Physicians

Amy Yasko, PhD, ND, NHD, AMD, HHP, FAAIM

& G.F. Gordon, MD, DO, MD(H)

This book is dedicated to Missie, Jessie, Cassie, Sloan, and Mark. Being blessed with healthy children is what inspires us to help others so that they may have the same gift and pure joy in their lives.

A special word of thanks are owed to Edward Yasko, Alexandra Van Cleve, Christine Blake, Nancy Guyon, Christopher Higgins, Andrew Raymond and everyone else who has assisted in the task of taking an individualized program and helping us to expand it into a generalized protocol.

Thank you to all the parents who share their stories of progress, hope, and yes, their setbacks on the AutismAnswer site. The concept of paying it forward has helped to make the site a haven for knowledge and hope. Special thanks to Erin, Michelle, Susan and Terri for the time they take on that site to help others.

We also thank all of the parents who have given us the privilege of helping their children to reach their full potential.

Contents

Foreword

May the life stories that are shared here and the testimonials throughout this book bring you peace in knowing that you are not alone on your journey towards the recovery of a loved one. Many have charted and stayed the course finding a reward that compares only to the miracle of life itself; a child who through the love of his family, returns from chaos to reach their full potential. We know the road is long, the way sometimes seems uncertain and the going can be tough. I truly wish that each person who takes up this book will benefit like those who have recovered their children and have become a symbol of hope for all of us.

With love and hope,
Dr. Amy

Michael's Story

Finding Dr. Amy

It was a cold day in February 2003. My son Michael was looking at the snow on the runway as we approached Metropolitan Detroit airport. Michael, now 8 years old, was diagnosed with autism in 1997 at the age of 20 months. We were returning from one of our many trips to cities around the United States. The search for help for Michael had been continuous for four years. We had been working through one DAN (Defeat Autism Now) Protocol treatment after another in hope of recovering Michael. During this period, we consulted with many competent and caring doctors, yet I knew our treatment plan was incomplete. For the previous eighteen months, we had been focusing on toxic metal chelation, and were not making any real progress. The chelating agents kept wreaking havoc on his gastro-intestinal tract causing constant starting, then stopping to treat GI dysbiosis, and then starting up again. I was determined to find another way!

I started searching for alternative chelation approaches, and as fate would have it, I discovered Dr. Garry Gordon's website. After reading several pages, I noticed that Dr. Gordon kept referring to Dr. Amy Yasko, a researcher and practitioner from Maine. After reading and re-reading everything on Amy's website, I was excited. I started to feel energized with renewed hope. Had I found someone who could take Michael to the next level? Would his path to recovery now run through Maine? The next day I phoned the office only to learn that it would take six to eight months to get started! Amy was becoming well known around the country for treating autism and many other inflammatory neurological disorders. A long waiting list had developed.

The Protocol

Finally, in June 2003, I received a call from Amy's husband Ed. Amy was ready to get started with Michael. I was a little apprehensive about starting because we had just committed Michael to a three-month stay in Atlanta. He was to begin a rigorous detoxification protocol at a well-known environmental medical clinic. I recalled how excited I was to discover Amy earlier in the year, and I was not going to miss out on this wonderful opportunity for Michael. We started both protocols simultaneously! I was very impressed by Amy's focus to detail in recording Michael's symptoms with me and in going over his files and files of lab results. Amy quickly customized a plan for Michael that was thorough, yet precise, and had a logical sequence to follow. The science behind her approach was convincing and the sequence just made good sense. The best part of all was that her plan for Michael was recovery. Anything less was unacceptable.

In reading this book, you will discover a great deal about the medical origin of your child's autism, how viruses and toxic metals result in excitotoxins causing devastation to the central nervous system, and how the brain can truly be healed after these toxins are removed. It is an intensive protocol that requires highly committed parents to be successful. I have found that combining Amy's protocol, with traditional laboratory testing and functional naturopathic monitoring, has worked very well for Michael. It has been extremely exciting and motivating to receive weekly lab results tracking excretion of toxic metals. Of equal importance, this protocol answers the tough question about what to do when the toxins have been removed and full recovery has not been achieved. For this difficult question, I am particularly grateful to Amy for step three entitled, “Program for Nerve Growth and Myelination”. This is where Michael is now. It is truly joyous to see our son re-emerge without the dreaded backward slides that we were accustomed to seeing.

Where We Are Today

The protocol has evolved and expanded significantly over the past year through careful monitoring of each child’s progress and through collaboration of Dr.Yasko with Dr. Gordon. We have made numerous adjustments in treatment intensity and type. Amy is never content to merely achieve recovery. She is constantly searching for ways to shorten the time frame.

As a result, Michael has made tremendous progress in recent months. Although his recovery is not yet complete, we are seeing daily improvements, causing much excitement at home and at school. For the first time, I can envision the complete and full return of our son from this horrific period in his and our lives.

I am confident that the protocol will continue to evolve, and rapidly. My advice to parents is to simply adopt this protocol and commit whatever is necessary to implement it. Never lose sight of the ultimate goal. Recovery! From the experienced “tried everything parents” to those dealing with a recent diagnosis, this book delivers a “how to” approach that gets results.

Robert Claeys
Ontario, Canada
June 2004

Dillon's Story

We have all been here.

Unless you are the parent of an autistic child, it is difficult to understand the harsh realities of trying to manage a son or daughter with this diagnosis. The constant day to day struggle to find foods that your child can eat, clothes that he can wear and places that you can take him to that are not too loud or too bright or too crowded and yet do not mind if your child needs to rock or spin in place or have screaming tantrums can seem like an overwhelming task. As the parent of an autistic child, you learn early that your child needs you to be caretaker, defender, investigator, and advocate to such an extent that you must give up the life you had before this child was born and build another one. A world where sleep no longer matters, where those first beautiful words from your child's mouth may never come, and where trips to the park or supermarket need to be managed with strategies worthy of an army general.

This is the life you build for yourself, until the day comes when you discover that there is a way out of this terrible prison, a journey which demands everything you have to give but grants miracles in return. Such a day came to me in June of 2004, with a phone call from Dr. Amy Yasko. After that moment, nothing would ever again be the same.

Dillon

My son, Dillon, was diagnosed with autism in 1994 at almost four years of age. As one of the early children affected by the autism epidemic, many doctors were still unfamiliar with remedies that might help him. I was told to seek a psychologist to help "manage" Dillon's behaviors as well as therapy for my family so that we could accept the stark reality of what we were about to face. There was little information then about helpful medical interventions for autism. Recommendations to follow a gluten-casein free diet came to me through special education personnel and not from our pediatrician. I instituted that diet when Dillon was six years old and noticed an immediate, positive improvement in his autistic behavior. Interestingly, few people then understood why the diet was effective. And it never occurred to me to question how a change in Dillon's food intake could curb his severe autistic behavior. I was only grateful that it did.

Through intensive therapies, including ABA, and the use of facilitated communication, Dillon was able to attend a regular elementary school, eventually winning scholarship awards and prizes for his poetry. As he continued to excel, I began to relax, feeling that Dillon was well on his way to becoming as independent as an autistic person could be.

But something was wrong with Dillon that went far beyond his autistic behaviors, something devastating to his health that I knew nothing about. By the time he was thirteen years old, he was almost six feet tall but weighed only 110 lbs. He was pale and gaunt and there were many types of foods that he could not eat because they affected his behavior drastically. His constant diarrhea meant a visit to our pediatrician several times a year but at each appointment I was told that "he would grow out of it." Finally, on the advice of a good friend, I found a doctor who could not only diagnosis Dillon's problem but offered evidence that his bowel condition could improve. Once given the diagnosis of autistic enterocolitis (a serious bowel condition), Dillon began taking a series of drugs to help his body heal. But each one only made him sicker and sicker until I began to wonder if this path to slow and uncertain recovery was worth the price he was paying. As time went on, it became clear that an alternative route to healing would have to be found for Dillon.

A way out

I went to Dr. Yasko because she was known as someone who handled "the hard cases" and was especially proficient with older children. After a lengthy discussion, she immediately pinpointed the problems with Dillon's medications and suggested other, more natural remedies that his body could absorb with greater ease. Three days after taking Dr. Yasko's advice, Dillon's therapy was under control and he began to feel relief from the terrible cramping pain that he had lived with for over twelve years.

With Dillon's genomic information as a starting point, Dr. Yasko then designed an individualized protocol for him using natural supplements, nucleotide drops and diet changes that took into account his specific genetic abnormalities. The building blocks used to create this specialized program are laid out in this book. As we added supplements and began to re-balance Dillon's system, the child who had disappeared behind the curtain of autism twelve years ago once again began to emerge. For the first time in years, Dillon was able to calm himself down as he gained more control over his anxiety levels and his motor functions. With time, he was also able to alleviate his constant obsessive-compulsive behaviors and impulsivity. Finally, and most exciting of all, he began to speak in an organized, meaningful way.

The protocol that you will read about in this book has changed my son's life in ways too numerous to mention. You will learn about the medical basis for the condition we now call "autism", which is not a static, genetically-caused disability, as we have been taught, but a collection of symptoms resulting from the inability of a fragile immune system to respond to our highly toxic environment. Gone are the days when we are required to accept this condition for our children. Dr. Yasko has created a treatment program that helps to eliminate these toxins from the body, allowing an affected child to recover into health.

Dillon continues to improve every day under Dr. Yasko's guidance. Although he has not yet completed the full detoxification program, he now weighs 165 pounds with much decreased abdominal distress and diarrhea; he skis, lifts weights and swims, all due to increased muscle tone and motor control; his academics have improved so much that he has time to work on writing his first novel; and, astonishingly, he speaks in short, simple sentences. No longer completely tied to his communication device, I foresee a day not too far into the future when Dillon will be able to attend college and perhaps, even graduate school. His life has been re-written thanks to Dr. Yasko and her highly effective treatments.

Dr. Yasko's Protocol

Only you can determine if this program will work for you and your child. As the co-founder of a non-profit corporation aimed at providing parents with much-needed information on biomedical interventions for autism, I have been exposed to a great deal of information about different treatment programs. After reviewing this information and speaking to literally hundreds of parents with autistic children, I can tell you that Dr. Yasko's protocol is one of the most comprehensive and effective of the many treatment programs now available. Through her extensive study of the underlying genomics which can lead to the condition we call autism, Dr. Yasko has uncovered the potential building blocks to achieving full recovery from this crippling diagnosis. No longer do we have to accept the life sentence that autism so often represents to the affected child and his family. If we are willing to march boldly forward, accepting that our children are sick and that treatments do exist to effectively manage this problem, we too can experience the miracle of recovery.

That is my wish for every one of you. That one day your child will be free from this terrible prison we call autism.

Julia York, M.A., J.D.
San Francisco, CA
March 2006

Preface

I feel privileged to participate in the development of this protocol for the full restoration of function for ALL autistic children - no matter how many other programs they may have already tried with varying degrees of success or failure. My colleague, Amy Yasko, with her background in molecular biology, immunology and infectious disease, is uniquely qualified to have developed a new perspective to this challenging disorder that continues to steal children away by the hundreds every single day.

My life's work has largely been centered around heavy metal detoxification. My website provides extensive documentation that everyone, child and adult, will have provable benefits by lowering their level of heavy metals through detoxification with oral chelation. Although I have been involved in trace mineral metabolism for over 35 years, there are always new developments that we must be aware of in dealing with today's proven levels of heavy metals and other pollutants that are now known to be adversely affecting the health of everyone on earth today. Some of these new developments are so powerful that they require a complete reevaluation of everything we thought we knew about the adverse effects of trace metals on our health. For example, we are faced with an epidemic of neurodegenerative diseases including Alzheimer's, ADD, ADHD, Multiple Sclerosis, ALS, etc. Heavy metals are clearly a major contributor to every one of these diseases. Autistic children are a case in point. After a lifetime of research in my field, my work with Dr. Amy Yasko has brought such radical new information to my attention that I am compelled (at age 69) to help re-educate the world, and help rewrite the textbooks on subjects like mercury and lead toxicity. This knowledge will help to bring effective therapies to the millions of patients around the world now afflicted with these neurodegenerative diseases.

Thanks to Dr. Yasko's work, we now have scientific validation that everything we thought we knew about heavy metals, and how to diagnose and treat these problems, was seriously deficient. She has patients where, according to the old rules, low levels of toxic metals in the urine after a provocative chelation challenge test should have indicated that further heavy metal detoxification for that patient would have been a complete waste of time and money. Dr. Yasko, with the help of dedicated parents, has found that negative urine-provoked tests for heavy metals may often mean nothing. She has demonstrated that RNA-based metal detoxification therapies can remove huge quantities of toxic metals from children who had received prior aggressive oral and/or parenteral chelation therapy with little or no benefit. The excellent results we are able to document have been achieved even after prolonged courses of DMSA or DMPS, frequently given by injection, had only marginal effects.

It is serendipity of the best kind that brought Dr. Yasko and I together at this point in our careers. We were both appointed to the board of NFAM (The National Foundation for Alternative Medicine) in Washington DC. We met at a dinner, and she started to tell me about the promising results she was getting in heavy metal detoxification using an oral EDTA based formula, the very product that I had formulated. When she began to tell me about the unbelievable increases in urine and fecal excretion of mercury, lead, antimony, cadmium etc. she was documenting using the Doctors Data Lab (whose work I have the greatest respect for), I had to learn more. She believed she was seeing these results because she had combined low doses of oral EDTA, Malic Acid and Garlic along with newly developed RNA products that when used properly are able to significantly lower the total body burden of pathogens. I knew then that we must work together.

Until that time, I was instructing all of the doctors doing chelation therapy that chelation therapy was only part of the treatment; getting the metals alone out was NOT enough, and in fact, effective chelation really requires a lifetime program because the earth is so polluted today. I had also emphasized the need to deal with the chronic levels of inflammation found today in virtually every chronic degenerative disease from cancer and heart disease to Alzheimer's disease. This inflammation has many contributors but it is due, in part, to chronic, low-grade infections in the body, which we now know that we all carry at all times throughout our life. Until I met and started to work with Dr. Yasko, my approach to dealing with both inflammation and pollution was so labor intensive, time consuming, and expensive that patients rarely adopted my comprehensive approach to achieving optimal health until cancer or another catastrophic disease was already present.

Dr. Yasko has one of the broadest views of anyone working in the field of autism. She understands that this disorder is a complicated puzzle and that full recovery requires an individualized approach - one that deals with each detail consistently over a prolonged timeframe. Dr. Yasko also understands that diet affects the activity of our genes and, as she has discovered, that nothing speaks as precisely to our genes as RNA, the molecule involved in cell-to-cell communication. Dr. Yasko is using RNA in this protocol to achieve levels of recovery in these children that may not have been possible otherwise.

However, I believe that the biggest use for RNA based research may not be as drugs, but as nutrients in new personalized nucleotide dietary supplement based programs using recently developed, unique, highly specific, extracted and purified nutritional products because of the information they can help convey.

The potential of RNA is validated by increased focus from a variety of areas within the scientific community. There are nearly 2000 new papers on RNA for medical indications published each year and over $2 billion has been spent worldwide by pharmaceutical companies trying to exploit the enormous potential of RNA. A recent article from Archives of Environmental Health, a publication for the National Institutes of Environmental Health, strongly states that research in RNA represents the most exciting development in biology of the decade, and that RNA research should lead to cures for cancer, AIDS, heart disease, ALS (amyotrophic lateral sclerosis), arthritis, etc.

In an article from the June 2004 issue of Discover, biochemist Jack Szostak hypothesizes that RNA based life may have existed before DNA based life and informs us "that the roles of the RNA in the cell have expanded beyond what any one imagined". RNA based therapies should be a key factor in helping develop the new paradigm of personalized medical practice to which the recently completed Human Genome Project must lead. Increased knowledge of our internal information network and the new gene expression microarray chips now being used in biomedical research will help us bypass the excessive current reliance on a pharmaceutical-based approach to medical care (see *Transducing the Genome* by Gary Zweiger). In fact, a new field of Bioinformatics is developing and information about millions of nucleotides is now stored in huge databases that the "new medicine" will be based on. It would appear that RNA's function might be as the "mother of all information networks."

This exciting new RNA technology will evolve into a convenient way to meet the need for preventive and health-promoting strategies for everyone, including safe and effective, documentable detoxification. Now we KNOW that autistic children, even those who are severely impaired, can completely recover. We are planning to develop a simplified version of this program for less severe problems (like ADD and ADHD, depression, OCD and other behavior or learning difficulties). Using this comprehensive RNA-based protocol for autism, a program that includes detoxification and lowering the pathogen burden, I see a way to improve the mental and physical health of every child. By supporting the body in every possible way, it is able to heal itself and lower its levels of various pathogens. When this occurs, the toxic metals that were locked inside cells are released in quantities never seen before in my years of working with trace minerals and chelation-centered heavy metal detoxification!

RNA based nutritional supplementation is the wave of the future, but we must recognize that giving RNA nutritional support without selecting what is appropriate for the particular needs of a patient will do some good and will clearly do no harm, but it is like playing all the 88 keys on the piano at the same time: you have sound but not music. I believe that the program we have put together for autism uses a variety of new specialized RNA based nucleotide dietary supplements to play the exact music these children need to hear in order to be well.

Dr. Garry Gordon
Payson, Arizona
July 7, 2004

The Motivation

"For years, Dr. Amy Yasko, an accomplished scholar, researcher, and clinician, has been quietly helping individuals recover from autism and other neurological disorders without drugs, injections, or other stressful, invasive procedures. As the parent of a child who has benefited greatly from Dr. Amy's expertise, I am delighted that Dr. Amy has written a book, which shares her blueprint for reversing autism with a wider audience. Parents and professionals seeking accessible, easy-to-implement, and most importantly, effective treatments for children or adults who are 'on the spectrum' will find this book to be an invaluable tool."

Mary W. Hopkins, Ed.D.
Mother of Alex, age 18

Autism is reaching epidemic proportions in this country and the world. Parents are desperately looking for answers. Physicians who work in this field are overwhelmed and often unable to help the older or the most severe children. There is an overwhelming need for a comprehensive approach to autism.

We have developed a protocol that has made a significant difference for a number of children of all ages, and all severities of autism. Word has spread about the success of our approach. We realized that in order to help each person who has contacted us, we needed to find a way to move from individualized programs to a more general protocol. Rather than taking another year to work on this book and explain every facet of this problem exhaustively, we have focused on what parents and practitioners really want — an approach that will work for all the doctors and parents who need it now.

We don't have the luxury of fully explaining every issue here. We realize you will need supplemental information. Our goal is to share our knowledge and results with you. We urge you to look at the additional resources section of the book. It will direct you to websites with newsletters, chat rooms, audio and videotapes and other written literature. We have included a section of sample data to give you specific information from children who have used this protocol. This is to help you understand that this is not a theory; it is a program that we have used and are continuing to use. We are not suggesting that it is a magic bullet; quite the contrary. The detailed protocol described in this book is not a cure all and it is not a quick fix. It takes time and patience.

No book can replace the individual consultations we have, or the customized programs we design for each child. This protocol is designed to assist each practitioner in his or her practice. The idea is to share a proven protocol and provide a basic understanding of the pieces involved. Helping these children requires a comprehensive approach; one that takes into account all of the pieces, not just a single piece of the complex puzzle of autism.

We have made an effort to acknowledge some of those outstanding individuals who have brought many of these individual pieces to light. We apologize in advance for failing to mention all of the others who work relentlessly to help bring all of these children back to health.

The Puzzle

"Prior to having worked with Dr. Amy, I thought that it was up to me and me alone to get my son well; but how? This was perhaps one of the most daunting aspects regarding his illness. During the past several months we have seen great progress with Mitch. One of the most important things I've come to realize is I do not have to do it alone! I have found an inner peace knowing that Mitch is on the road to recovery. Together, Dr. Amy and I are working to get my child well."

Margaret Wilson
Mother of Mitch, age 7

Sometimes a number of seemingly unrelated events occur simultaneously resulting in disaster. A prime example of this was the death of Princess Diana. If she had been wearing her seatbelt, if the car hadn't been speeding, if the driver hadn't been drinking, if the paparazzi weren't chasing the car...eliminate any one of those factors and a tragedy might have been averted. The multitude of factors that must occur to create the condition we call "autism" can be viewed in a similar fashion.

If an MTHFr mutation was not present, if there was less of a heavy metal burden, if there was no chronic viral infection, if no underlying streptococcal infection existed, if we didn't have excitotoxin damage... the negative cascade of neurological events that ends in a spectrum disorder may not have happened. So autism can be viewed as the puzzle, created from these various biochemical, genetic and physiological factors all careening together in the body of a developing child. To make informed decisions about undoing the damage that has been done in this "crash" of negative factors, each piece of this puzzle must be examined carefully, its function understood, and balance restored.

This book will look at each piece of this puzzle, as we understand it at this time, and suggest supplementation programs to address potential imbalances. The information presented reflects the most current view of the process of neurological inflammation that results in "autistic-like" behaviors, including the entire spectrum of autism-related diseases. This field is evolving almost daily with new information and new literature, and we will evolve with it. We expect that there will be additions, modifications and revisions to this book as new information comes to light.

There is not yet complete agreement between your authors on every detail in the proposed treatment plans (like all doctors, we are greatly influenced by what has worked for our patients). But the two of us bring well over sixty years of combined experience, and a passion for finding answers for what have seemed to be impossible problems (always utilizing the least toxic and most natural approaches) to the enormous challenge of autism. We will not give up until every child is given the chance to recover; until all of the pieces of the puzzle fit together, and this chronic disease no longer threatens the next generation.

This protocol cannot answer every question with regard to autism or other types of neurological inflammation. This is a starting point and we envision that individuals who are following this protocol will take advantage of the website www.autismanswer.com. This site will continue this initial effort, permitting questions and answers from health professionals learning to use this protocol, and another discussion group separately for parents working with this protocol. This protocol does, however, provide an explanation for many of the observed behaviors and symptoms that are associated with autism; a framework from which to help reverse many of these traits, and a rationale for why many of the currently utilized therapies are effective.

Understanding the Individual Pieces

"After 2 years of taking our son to Doctors around the US that address one area of the complicated biomedical puzzle called autism, we were fortunate enough to find Dr. Amy. Dr. Amy examined all the pieces of our son's chemistry, not just one. She didn't try to fit him into a shoe that didn't fit, but created one for him that did fit. Our very affected son made more progress in 2 months working with Dr. Amy than he had made in the last 2 years. He continues to improve before our eyes. Dr. Amy has given hope back to us. She has helped us to begin to reclaim our son and our life."

Dave & Jennifer Larson
Parents to Cade, age 3 ½

In autistic individuals, imbalances have been shown to occur in a number of organ systems, neurotransmitters, and biochemical processes in the body. These include excess excitotoxins, heavy metal toxicity, methylation deficiencies, chronic viral and bacterial infections, fluctuations in serotonin, norepinephrine and dopamine, and liver, pancreas, stomach, intestinal, adrenal, thyroid and hormonal imbalances.

It is possible to rebalance all of these systems. This is true for any child with autism; there is no magic age or age limitation for this approach. However this is a process, it is a marathon, not a sprint. It takes time and patience. Success can be achieved by calmly correcting each imbalance. We liken this effort to the years of effort and expense some go through in restoring a classic car to its show room elegance. We are convinced that tremendous brainpower is present in autistic children and we are dedicated to helping them let it shine.

Excitotoxins

Excitotoxins will continue to damage more nerves and wreak more havoc in the body if they are not addressed. Therefore the excitotoxin imbalance is the best place to start to put the pieces back together. Once excitotoxins are under control, it is easier to balance the rest of the body. This is an area where we encounter disagreement with some of our colleagues. The reason we are holding to our approach is that we have been able to help children who were not helped by approaches that ignored the vital role of excitotoxins in inflammation. Due to a basic lack of understanding about the involved chemistry, we find that glutamic acid, glutamine, etc. are still being included in supplement regimes for their potential gastro-intestinal benefits, while their documented potential for contributing to the proven neurotoxic effects are being ignored. Every decision needs to be based on potential benefits vs. potential risks.

Over seven years ago, Dr. Russell Blaylock described the pathway of excitotoxin damage and the role it plays in neurological damage brilliantly in his landmark book on excitotoxins. He spelled out specifically how and why MSG, hydrolyzed vegetable protein, aspartame and related compounds have been proven to cause death of neurons beyond any reasonable doubt. More recently, this concept of excitotoxin damage has been found to pertain to autism. Excitotoxins are neurotransmitters such as glutamate or aspartate that can excite the nerves to death when their levels are not regulated properly. Foods or supplements that contain excitotoxins include MSG (monosodium glutamate), glutamic acid, glutamine, NutraSweet, aspartate, aspartame, and cysteine. Mercury and aluminum can trigger glutamate release. Minimizing glutamate is a differentiating factor in our protocol and has helped many autistic children significantly. Since our goal is to help ALL patients we believe this extra aspect of neurological disease must be recognized if we are going to provide the maximum potential benefits to our children.

Glutamate is the main excitatory neurotransmitter in the body. It is essential for learning and for both short-term and long-term memory. It is also the precursor to the inhibitory neurotransmitter, GABA. GABA is a calming neurotransmitter, and is essential for speech. GABA neurons damp the propagation of sounds so that a distinction can be made between the onset of a sound and background noise. (GABA is often used to help restore speech in individuals who have suffered strokes.) Problems occur if the normal process of regulation of glutamate malfunctions and if toxic levels of this excitatory neurotransmitter build up in the synaptic junctions.

The balance between glutamate and GABA is like a seesaw. Under normal conditions, when the glutamate side gets too high, the GABA side of the seesaw will increase and decrease the glutamate. Under normal functioning conditions, excess levels of the excitotoxin glutamate will convert to GABA. There seems to be a "disconnect" in this process for autistic children so that the excitatory neurotransmission is high (stims) and the calming neurotransmission is low (lack of speech). When conditions occur that throw off this delicate balance, then high levels of glutamate can accumulate while the levels of GABA remain exceedingly low. This would create a situation that would require decreasing the glutamate levels, and increasing the GABA levels in order to restore balance. Chronic viral infection (there is increasing evidence that all of us suffer from one or more of these chronic infections throughout most of our lifetimes) may be related to this disconnect between glutamate and GABA.

Acute viral infection can lead to Type I diabetes. In Type I diabetes the body makes antibodies against the enzyme that converts glutamate to GABA, leading to a "disconnect" between glutamate and GABA regulation. It is tempting to speculate that if acute viral infection can cause this disconnect, it is possible that chronic viral infection can also lead to a similar disconnect between glutamate and GABA regulation. One final note on this conversion from glutamate to GABA is that the enzyme that is responsible for the conversion, GAD (glutamic acid decarboxylase) uses vitamin B6 as a cofactor for its activity. The use of B6 for autism is a longstanding part of the DAN treatment, pioneered by Dr. Bernard

Rimland. It is possible that B6 has been acting to aid in the conversion of glutamate to GABA in addition to its other roles in the body.

Once this disconnect has occurred, the brain requires sufficient levels of oxygen and energy to remove excess glutamate. However, glutamate release leads to the release of insulin, which results in decreased glucose levels. The amount of glucose in the brain regulates the removal of excess glutamate from the synapses. Therefore, a drop in blood glucose disrupts this removal process and allows the build up of toxic glutamate. In fact, conditions of hypoglycemia, or low calorie/starvation conditions induce the release of glutamate and reduce the ability to remove excess levels of glutamate from the brain. This excess glutamate depletes glutathione. Glutathione is one of the most powerful antioxidants found in the body and helps to protect neurons from damage. Glutathione depletion consequently leads to the death of additional neurons.

Glutamate has six different types of receptors to which it can bind in the brain. One of these receptors, the NMDA receptor, is tied to calcium transport as its mode of action. In the case of the NMDA receptors, the release of excess glutamate triggers an inflammatory cascade that results in the death of neurons by the major influx of calcium into the nerve until it results in neural cell death. Normal levels of calcium result in normal neuron functioning. However, excessive levels of calcium make it impossible for the neuron to rest; the neuron continues to fire without stopping, causing the release of inflammatory mediators, the release of more glutamate, thus resulting in more calcium influx. The high intracellular levels of calcium also lead to high levels of nitric oxide and peroxynitrite, causing damage to the energy producing apparatus of the cells. Magnesium (a second part of Dr. Rimland's protocol) is able to modulate the calcium flow, as is zinc. However, zinc is a double-edged sword as it is also able to activate glutamate release via the non-NMDA glutamate receptors.

Although these receptors are called "glutamate receptors", any of the excitatory amino acids are able to bind to the receptors and cause excitotoxin damage. The toxic potential of these excitatory amino acids has been suggested to be proportional to their ability to excite neurons. These excitatory amino acids include glutamate, aspartate and to a lesser extent, cysteine and homocysteine.

Glutamate and aspartate are common as food additives as well as naturally occurring components of a large number of foods. In cells, glutamate and aspartate can be synthesized from each other. In the presence of ATP, glutamine will convert to glutamate. The two main food additives that are sources for excitotoxins are MSG (monosodium glutamate) and aspartame (NutraSweet). High levels of glutamate and aspartate are found naturally in protein rich foods, including very high levels in wheat gluten, and milk casein. The process of making protein into a protein powder releases glutamate from its bound form, resulting in the ingestion of free unbound glutamate. While these amino acids are necessary for normal brain function, excess amounts of them create a wide range of bodily damage. Body systems that have been affected by glutamate toxicity include effects on white blood cells (elevations in the levels of eosinophils), effects on blood vessels (causing migraines and reduced regulation of blood pressure), and inhibition of the conversion of glutamate to GABA. Excess glutamate can cause vestibular dysfunction resulting in nystagmus. The sites in the brain that have been reported to be damaged by excitotoxins include the hypothalamus, the hippocampal neurons, and the Purkinje neurons, among others.

The recent finding that copper suppresses GABA ties together disruptions in copper/zinc ratios in the body to glutamate and GABA imbalances, which is yet another piece of the puzzle. These disruptions in zinc/copper ratios have been well characterized by Dr. William Walsh of the Pfeiffer Clinic. (Yet another piece of this complex puzzle comes into play, the successful use of EDTA as a standard in the supplement program of autistic children. EDTA will help to decrease copper levels. This will release the GABA from copper suppression, and will help to rebalance the zinc/copper ratio).

There has been a suggestion of a relationship between heavy metal toxicity and glutamate in the literature. As referenced in Aschner et al "In the absence of glutamate, neurons are unaffected by acute exposure to mercury, suggesting that neuronal dysfunction is secondary to disturbances in astrocytes." And "Co-application of nontoxic concentrations of methylmercury and glutamate leads to the typical appearance of neuronal lesions associated with excitotoxic stimulation." (Methylmercury alters glutamate transport in astrocytes. Neurochem Int. 2000; 37:199) this would suggest that lower concentrations of mercury might be more toxic in the presence of excess glutamate or other excitotoxins.

Excess levels of glutamate have been implicated in a range of neurodegenerative diseases, including Alzheimer's disease, Parkinson's disease, Huntington's chorea, stroke, Multiple sclerosis, and ALS. In the case of autism, irregularities related to glutamate have been observed. In addition, glutamate, glutamic acid and aspartate and aspartic acid were found to be elevated in individuals exhibiting autistic behavior relative to controls.

Children with autistic type behavior have often been described as exceedingly intelligent, even to the extreme point of being considered savants in particular areas. Dr. Tsien and his collaborators have demonstrated a correlation between glutamate receptors and superior ability in learning and memory. By overproducing a component of one of the glutamate receptors, they were able to increase the level of glutamate binding. This was the first demonstration of a relationship between increased glutamate/ glutamate receptors and higher intelligence. The down side of the enhanced level of glutamate was an increased risk of stroke and seizure activity. This work suggests a potential correlation between intelligence and glutamate levels. It also points to the potential increased susceptibility to excitotoxin damage due to excess glutamate/glutamate receptor activity as a consequence of enhanced intelligence.

While there have been reports that the density of glutamate receptors is decreased in autism, this may be due to receptor recycling as a function of glutamate binding rather than an actual lack of receptors. Cells are constantly in the process of selecting and recycling receptors. Recycling occurs, and is more complex in neurons. In neurons recycling is complicated by the fact that internalized proteins have the possibility of returning to their surface of origin or to a second plasma membrane domain. This would seem likely in this case, for although the receptor density was decreased, the mRNA levels of glutamate receptors were significantly increased in autism.

Regardless of the reasons for the glutamate excess in autism, it is a critical first step to remove excitotoxin triggers from the diet. This involves reading labels and closely monitoring food and supplement intake to avoid excitotoxins. The Appendix of this book contains a list of excitotoxins and the other names by which they are known.

The Liver

The liver is one of the most important organs in terms of maintaining health. It is the site for carbohydrate, fat and protein metabolism, storage of vitamins and minerals, and regulatory mechanisms for blood sugar and hormone levels. Bile production, which is necessary for elimination reactions, also takes place in the liver. In addition, and perhaps most importantly, the liver is the site for detoxification of the body. A central problem in the treatment of autism is the function and health of the liver. If the liver is healthy, it can make sufficient enzymes for the efficient detoxification of the body.

The liver contains high levels of enzymes that are required for detoxification processes. It contains one of the highest levels of glutathione, one of the most powerful antioxidants found in the body. Glutathione is essential for both the Phase I and Phase II detoxification systems of the liver. Phenol-sulphotransferase (PST) is another sulfur-containing enzyme that detoxifies leftover hormones and toxic molecules, as well as food dyes and chemicals. Metallothionein are sulfur-containing proteins that scavenge free radical and regulate metals. In the case of autistic children, almost 100% have low PST enzyme levels. Both the PST enzymatic detoxification systems, as well as glutathione require sulfur. The metallothioneins, MT proteins that are involved in heavy metal detoxification in the body, are also sulfur-containing proteins. This lack of sulfur seems to be a central problem with children exhibiting autistic behavior.

High extra-cellular levels of the excitotoxin glutamate cause the extrusion of intracellular cysteine resulting in glutathione depletion. Low levels of magnesium also result in decreased levels of glutathione, as does infection or inflammation that causes elevations in TNF alpha. Heavy metal toxicity may be exacerbated due to the lack of sulfur/glutathione detoxification systems; this heavy metal toxicity then triggers further excitotoxin release, which creates a continuous cycle of inflammation and depletion of antioxidants and detoxification proteins.

The function and health of the liver and pancreas appear to be at the center of many of the health issues seen in these children. While sulfur-containing supplements are useful as chelating agents, they are also serving to supply sulfur for glutathione, the PST enzyme system, for taurine, and as antioxidants.

The Stomach, Pancreas, and Intestinal Tract

In an ideal situation, following the digestion of food in the stomach by hydrochloric acid, the HCL is dumped into the small intestine stimulating the release of several proteins. These proteins include gastric inhibitory peptide (GIP), secretin, and cholecystokinin (CCK). GIP slows the release of acid into the intestinal tract, secretin stimulates the pancreas to release bicarbonate to neutralize the acid, and CCK stimulates the gall bladder to release the bile (made by the liver) into the intestines to neutralize the acid and help digest fats. In addition, GABA release may help to reduce the triggering of transient lower esophageal relaxations, decreasing gastroesophageal reflux (GERD). GABA is also essential for proper intestinal motility. If, however, the pancreas and the liver are in a weakened state, this ideal situation will not occur. Instead, the HCL is still dumped into the small intestine, but these three proteins will not be released properly. This results in a situation where the intestinal tract becomes more acidic due to lack of released bile, and results in an environment that is more conducive to growth of microorganisms. The resulting microorganisms in the intestinal tract may contain a wide variety of anaerobic bacteria, including a number of species of *Clostridium.* In addition, there will be an overgrowth of yeast, *Eschericia coli*, and *Streptococcus*, rather than normal intestinal flora.

James Russell, a professor in the Section of Microbiology at Cornell University, Senior Research Microbiologist of the USDA, and a recognized expert in *E.coli* has stated that, *"Escherichia coli* is a common bacterium in the GI tract, but it is usually outnumbered by other types. *E. coli* is never a beneficial bacterium, but under normal circumstances the animal and *E. coli* tolerate each other. Some strains of *E. coli*, however, are not people-friendly, and these highly virulent forms can cause acute illness or even death."

In addition to creating imbalances in intestinal flora, an added result of insufficient bile relative to acid will be inadequate digestion of fats, consequently a decrease in absorption of fat-soluble nutrients (i.e. vitamins A, D, and K); and a sub-optimal amount of secretin and CCK to trigger communication with the brain. Decreased levels of CCK in the brain are correlated with anxiety and panic. There are also indications that adequate CCK levels are important in addressing microbial infection in the body.

Secretin has been shown to potentiate the levels of CCK induced enzymes, and this may be an additional benefit associated with its use. Similar to CCK, the hormone secretin is found in the brain as well as the GI tract. Secretin has been shown to cross the blood/brain barrier. It is postulated that secretin that crosses over into the brain as well as secretin that is released by Purkinje cells in the brain may regulate cells nearby to produce GABA.

Neuropeptide Y is another peptide that is abundant in both the brain and the GI tract. In the brain it is involved in regulation of appetite, anxiety and blood pressure. In the GI tract Neuropeptide

Y is involved in the regulation of pancreatic secretions and gut motility. Neuropeptide Y has been reported to suppress glutamate and antagonize the effects of glutamate.

Glucagon-like peptide is another gut peptide that is involved in associative and spatial learning and memory, and also involved in neuro protection from glutamate-induced damage.

Gluten and casein free diets have been found to be helpful in autistic children. Wheat, casein, and hydrolyzed yeast are concentrated sources of glutamate. Wheat gluten is 43% glutamate and milk casein is 23% glutamate. Consequently, a diet that is high in casein, gluten, and yeast would exacerbate a system that is already overwhelmed with excess excitotoxins. However, the milk protein casein and whey are powerful stimulators of CCK. Diets deficient in casein and whey could lead to further imbalances in CCK levels in the GI tract, necessitating additional stimuli for CCK.

On a related note, endocannabinoid synthesis is triggered in the brain as a protective response to excitotoxin damage. This protective release of endogenous cannabinoids could lead to elevated levels of opioids. These endocannabinoids in the brain also suppress the release of both CCK and GABA, further decreasing their levels.

The role of the pancreas in the conversion of glutamate to GABA has already been discussed. The pancreas is a critical piece of the autism puzzle. If the pancreas is not healthy the result can be high glutamate levels, low GABA levels, decreased secretin, decreased CCK, and decreased Vitamin K, among other imbalances.

Vitamin K Deficiency

Excess stomach acid and insufficient bile (due to decreased liver function) creates a situation of relative acid excess and acid pH in the intestinal tract. (Ingestion of glutamate as MSG itself has been reported to cause excess acid and heartburn.) This would create an environment that is conducive to yeast, *E.coli*, and *streptococcal* overgrowth and non-ideal for normal protective bacterial flora. This imbalance in normal flora can be further exacerbated by the excitotoxin glutamate. Excess glutamate has been shown to increase the survival of enterohemorrhagic *E.coli*, particularly under acidic conditions.

While Vitamin K is a fat-soluble vitamin, it is not stored like the other fat-soluble vitamins; consequently it needs to be absorbed on a daily basis. Normally this occurs when the bacteria in the GI tract process leafy greens. If however, the normal flora of the GI tract has been disturbed there will be a Vitamin K deficiency. Most likely all children are born deficient in Vitamin K, as it does not cross the placenta.

Vitamin K is essential for healthy calcium metabolism, and has functions related to blood clotting. It prevents excessive bruising and bleeding; is important for strong bone and teeth health; and for sugar regulation (controlling hypoglycemic-related anxiety attacks). It has also been shown that Vitamin K2 can help prevent pathologic accumulations of calcium in tissue, which we will learn is one of the critical factors leading to cell death. One of the highest levels of vitamin K in the body is in the pancreas, which is critical for sugar regulation in the body. Most children suffering from autistic behavior seem to have imbalances in their ability to tolerate sugars. In addition to the brain, the other area of the body that is able to concentrate the excitotoxin glutamate is the pancreas, which would result in further damage to the pancreas and sugar regulation.

Vitamin K reacts enzymatically with glutamate and calcium to ensure proper placement of the calcium in bones and teeth. In addition, Vitamin K is a cofactor for the conversion of glutamate to gamma carboxyglutamate. Lack of vitamin K would then create a cycle of deregulation in the glutamate/calcium pathway leading to further neurological inflammation.

Streptococcal Infection

Dr. Vojdani, Dr. Bock and their colleagues have demonstrated the presence of antibodies to Streptococcal M protein, as well as autoantibodies against neuron-specific antigens in blood samples taken from autistic children. Under certain conditions, antibodies targeted against the basal ganglia of the brain have been found to follow *streptococcal* infection. *Streptococcal* infection has been implicated in leaky gut syndrome, as well as a wide variety of behavioral disturbances given the acronym PANDAS (Pediatric Autoimmune Neuropsychiatric Disorders Associated with Streptococcal infections) that have been described by Dr. Susan Swedo. In addition, Dr. Maddie Hornig and Dr. Ian Lipkin and their colleagues (Hoffman et al) have developed an animal model of *streptococcal* infection that results in motor and behavioral disturbances.

Streptococcal infection is known to lead to elevated levels of the inflammatory cytokines NFKB and TNF alpha. High levels of TNF alpha have been implicated in Tourettes syndrome, facial tics, obsessive-compulsive behavior, and schizophrenia. In addition, the level of TNF alpha is inversely correlated with glutathione levels. Consequently, high TNF alpha levels as a result of *streptococcal* infection would result in decreases in glutathione levels.

Generally, bacteria elicit a B cell mediated immune response, and viruses elicit a T cell mediated immune response. However, *streptococci*, all of which have the ability to nonspecifically stimulate T cells, elaborate a large number of extra-cellular toxins. Therefore, once an immune response is mounted against *streptococcus* it would involve both T cell and B cells resulting in a major inflammatory reaction. A chronic *streptococcal* infection could therefore lead to a depletion of both T and B cell mediated immune factors. Conversely, an inadequate T and/or B cell response to *streptococci* could result in chronic underlying *streptococcal* infection.

Streptococci are also known to elicit a number of other factors in addition to these toxins. These factors include streptokinase (which increases the inflammatory mediators TNF alpha and IL6), neuraminidase (which can aid in the establishment of viral infections), and NADase (which depletes NAD that is necessary for recycling of glutathione), and glutathione peroxidase (necessary for virulence).

Chronic *streptococcal* infections (i.e. ear infections) and the use of easily abused antibiotics (as noted in the book *The Killers Within:*

The Deadly Rise of Drug Resistant Bacteria) that follows can result in a lack of re-population of the intestines with normal flora with a subsequent loss of Vitamin K. Consequently, the net results of *streptococcal* infection are depletion of Vitamin K levels, decreased glutathione levels, potential over-stimulation followed by depletion of the immune system, increased TNF alpha levels (which trigger OCD, facial tics, etc.), potential autoimmune responses and inflammatory reactions against various areas of the body including the heart, the basal ganglia and the GAGs in the GI tract.

Streptococcus may permanently reside as part of the bacteria or flora in the nasopharyngeal cavity of children who are highly susceptible to *streptococci*. The mucous system in our nasal passages flushes bacteria and viruses into our stomach. It is easy to see how under "compromised conditions", *streptococci* could survive the stomach and make its way to the intestinal tract. Gastric reflux has been implicated as a factor in ear infections. (Gastric reflux may be associated with low levels of GABA.) It is not surprising then to note that in addition to its role in ear infections and strep throat, *streptococcus* has been implicated in leaky gut. Gut flora changes play a major role in causing the increased intestinal membrane permeability that is seen with leaky gut. Depletion of glutathione is a common occurrence in leaky gut. *Streptococcal* infection, or the presence of chronic or recent infection, depletes glutathione levels. High glutamate levels also result in the depletion of glutathione. *Streptococcal* infection is also more likely to be an issue in individuals with high glutamate levels, as glutamate is related to virulence in *streptococci*. *Streptococcus* flourishes in a high glutamate, low glutathione environment. Thus, the combined effects of changes in gut flora and depleted glutathione lay the groundwork for leaky gut.

We know that if a child eats the same foods too frequently, the leaky gut will lead to that child's reacting badly to even the few foods that manage to survive the "do not eat list" that they seemed to tolerate well initially. With all these limitations, when we finally find something that our child likes, the danger is that we rely on it excessively. Until we have healed the intestine, the body can

both sulfur donors as well as lipid based support. Part of the reason for this intolerance to sulfur support, including high dose sulfur based chelation, is that a net result of CBS up regulations is that intermediates of the methylation cycle are converted to toxic sulfur byproducts by increased activity in the subsequent step of the pathway. When sulfur groups are tied up in amino acids such as homocysteine, methionine, SAMe, SAH, or cysteine, the sulfur is not free to create havoc in the system. By virtue of increased CBS activity, these sulfur groups that were complexed (or tied up) as part of the methylation cycle in the form of amino acids, are now released into the system as sulfites which are toxic to the body and deplete much needed molybdenum from the system. A similar situation exists with respect to amino groups and the generation of ammonia. A quote from Ingenblee and Young (Nutrition Research Reviews, December 2004) helps to eloquently describe this relationship *"Adaptive conservation of N and S body stores is reached by a functional restraint of the trans-sulfuration cascade, through the depression of cystathionine -synthase activity (CBS). As a result, upstream accumulation of homo-cysteine favors its re-methylation conversion to methionine which helps maintain metabolic path-ways of survival value."*

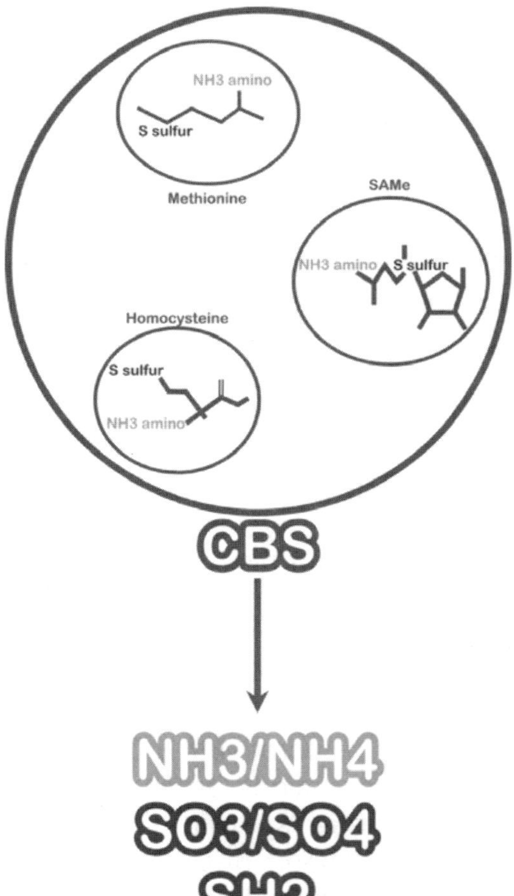

Methylation is related to neurotransmitter levels. Methylation of intermediates tryptophan metabolism can affect the levels of serotonin. Intermediates of the methylation pathway are also shared with the pathway involved in dopamine synthesis. Consequently, imbalances or supplementation of the methylation pathway will also affect the neurotransmitter dopamine. In addition to its direct role as a neurotransmitter, dopamine is involved in methylating phospholipids in the cell membranes, and has been extensively described by Dr. Richard Deth. This methylation of phospholipids helps to keep the cell membranes fluid. Membrane fluidity is important for a variety of reasons including proper signaling of the immune system as well as protecting nerves from damage. The role of membrane fluidity in nerve damage has been described in ALS and Alzheimer's disease.

Increases in certain inflammatory mediators, such as IL6 and TNF alpha, lead to decreases in methylation. Chronic inflammation would therefore exacerbate an existing genetic condition of undermethylation. The inability to progress normally through the methylation pathway, can lead to a build up of precursors of the methylation pathway, including the excitotoxin glutamate.

This altered methylation cycle activity can lead to low levels of DNA and RNA synthesis, as the building blocks for DNA and RNA require the methylation pathway. This makes it difficult for the body to synthesize new cells. This would result in a decreased level of new T cell synthesis. *De novo* T cell synthesis is necessary to respond to viral infection, as well as for other aspects of the proper functioning of the immune system. T cells are necessary for antibody producing cells in the body (B cells) as both T helpers and T suppressors to appropriately regulate the antibody response.

In addition, the decreased level of methylation can result in improper DNA regulation. DNA methylation is necessary to <u>prevent</u> the expression of viral genes that have been inserted into the body's DNA. Loss of methylation can lead to the <u>expression</u> of inserted viral genes.

Proper levels of methylation are also directly related to the body's ability to both myelinate nerves and to "prune" nerves.

Myelin is a sheath that wraps around the neuronal wiring to insulate and facilitate faster transmission of electrical potentials. Without adequate methylation, the nerves cannot myelinate in the first place or cannot remyelinate after insults such as viral infection or heavy metal toxicity. A secondary effect of a lack of methylation, hence decreased myelination, is inadequate "pruning" of nerves. Pruning helps to prevent excessive wiring, or unused neural connections, and reduces the synaptic density. Without adequate pruning the brain cell connections are misdirected and proliferate into dense, bunched thickets. There is literature (Nature Neuroscience, Vol 7 April 2004) suggesting that proper myelination is necessary to ensure the subsequent pruning of nerves.

Inadequate myelination and pruning of nerves as a result of decreased methylation may relate to the published MRI results of Dr. Martha Herbert. She has reported that the outer area of white matter in the brain was larger in autistic children than in controls, while the inner zones of white matter were not different. According to Dr. Herbert, the outer zone that showed the increase in volume is the area that myelinates later; this may help to elucidate a timeline for problems in myelination and pruning.

Heavy Metals

The toxic effects of heavy metals, including mercury, have been well characterized and documented by Dr. Amy Holmes and Dr. Stephanie Cave, among others. The heavy metal burden of our children is now being openly acknowledged by the EPA in their statements that over 600,000 babies are born each year with elevated levels of mercury. The sources of this mercury are ubiquitous since we release over 600 tons of mercury into the air annually just from burning coal for our electric power. Although autistic children do NOT usually reveal significant levels in their hair (since they appear to have a defect in their ability to detoxify mercury), they, like everyone on the planet, carry far higher levels of all toxic heavy metals than any humans did as recently as 400 years ago. Lead also averages 1000 times higher concentration in all human bones tested anywhere on earth today than four centuries ago. Levels of lead, mercury and cadmium are all found to be in far greater concentrations than what is recommended for optimal health and longevity. These heavy metals are contributing to the epidemic of degenerative disease we are seeing today in every country in all age groups.

Toxic metals accumulate in our bodies over our lifetimes beginning with the amounts we receive from our mothers during pregnancy, metals we are inoculated with during vaccination, and the metals we consume and breath every day thereafter. Dr. David Steinman and Dr. Samuel Epstein have written a comprehensive guide to the toxins in our daily lives that add to this total body toxic burden.

Many of the symptoms seen in autism resemble aspects of heavy metal toxicity. A number of treatment protocols for autism include metal chelation and detoxification and have proven successful in helping to reverse symptoms of autism. We have chosen not to use intravenous chelation agents whenever possible, rather to focus primarily on the use of oral and topically administered EDTA as our primary heavy metal chelator.

An important part of the protocol presented in this book includes a proprietary approach to metal detoxification that allows us to target metals that may be sequestered by virus as well as bacteria in the body. We discovered that none of the available chelators eliminate these "bound" metals, so we developed a unique, oral, RNA-based process to work in conjunction with a supplement based program to aid the body in dealing with these chronic infections. We are pleased with the success that this new approach is providing and see clinical improvements along with significant increases in urine and/or fecal excretion of toxic metals. These results suggest to us that these chronic infections have been efficiently binding toxic metals in the body where no chelating agent seems to be able to effectively remove them. We have seen these results even with patients who have undergone extensive parenterally administered DMPS, to the point that others had been convinced that mercury was no longer an issue. Even in these previously treated patients, we are finding substantial releases of mercury as well as other toxic metals as the viral and bacterial load is reduced. With this elimination of virus, bacteria and toxic metals, we have also seen patients' symptoms improve dramatically.

A mechanism by which chronic viral infection may lead to the observed retention of heavy metals involves host metallothionein proteins. Viruses have been shown to induce the synthesis of host metallothionein proteins (MT). MT proteins help to detoxify heavy metals including mercury, and to balance zinc and copper in the body. It is documented that viral infection can cause an increase in the level of MT proteins that is directed by the virus. MT proteins that are triggered in response to viral infection are able to bind the heavy metals in the body. However, unlike MT proteins that are made in response to cellular signals, these viral-triggered MT may act to sequester the metals inside the cell. It is important to remember that viruses are parasites; they are not free-living organisms. It is in the best interest of the virus to keep "the host" (in this case the child) immuno-compromised so that the virus continues to have a home. If the virus were able to aid in trapping heavy metals inside the cells, it would certainly help to keep the host immuno-compromised. This later association of MT proteins, virus and heavy metals might also help to explain the lack of available host MT proteins in autistic children described by Dr. Bill Walsh. If viral infection has commandeered host MT synthesis, it would result in the observed decrease in host MT levels. If this is in fact the scenario, then it would help to explain the difficulty in removing heavy metals from autistic children. It would be necessary to eliminate chronic virus in order to fully eradicate heavy metals from the body.

In an analogous fashion, bacteria have been shown to accumulate the toxic metal aluminum. It might be anticipated that addressing chronic bacterial infection in the body would be necessary to see the excretion of aluminum from the system. Preliminary data presented by Dr. Yasko suggests that this is in fact the case. Programs that help to support the elimination of chronic bacterial infection from the body, also illicit the excretion of aluminum in the urine.

There are a number of agents that are currently utilized for chelation of heavy metals including DMSA, DMPS, EDTA, glutathione, alpha lipoic acid, and garlic. Each of these agents has antiviral capabilities. Garlic is well known as an antiviral, antifungal, antibacterial nutritional supplement. Glutathione is one of the body's most important defense mechanisms against viruses. There are examples in the literature of EDTA eliciting virus from cells. DMSA, which is widely held as solely a mercury chelator, has been described to have antiviral activity; more specifically anti-retroviral activity (measles and mumps are retroviruses). DMSA is commonly used to help to chelate heavy metals and for detoxification with children exhibiting autistic behavior. However, it is important to realize that DMSA has been shown to trigger the inflammatory mediator TNF alpha so it would be important to use caution and to actively add agents that effectively can reduce and/or control inflammation when using DMSA. (We have been able to accomplish this anti-inflammatory effect consistently and conveniently in all of our patients with an RNA-based oral liquid product that is easily added to the treatment program of all children, since it can even be added to their food.) DMPS is also listed on the NIAID therapeutics database as showing antiviral activity against HIV. Both DMSA and DMPS have potential side effects and should be used with caution and under the care of a doctor familiar with chelation protocols.

It is possible that all of these chelating agents act to both chelate heavy metals as well as to trigger chronic virus containing metals from the body. The "detox rash" that most parents of autistic children are familiar with, may actually be in part a viral rash, as chronic virus is eliminated from the body.

RNA Viruses

The positive rationale behind vaccination is to prevent more serious disease from active, acute, naturally-acquired infections. Natural acute measles, mumps and rubella infections have been known to have potentially serious repercussions including brain damage, deafness, and blindness and photosensitivity, in addition to neurotoxicity.

The particular combination of viruses used in the MMR vaccine is unique in that all three are single-stranded RNA viruses. Measles and mumps are negative-stranded RNA retroviruses, and rubella is a positive-stranded RNA virus. Human cells do not contain enzymes for copying their own RNA. As a result, the viruses bring in their own enzymes with them in order to initiate replication once they have infected a cell. The virus diverts the host's (the human cells) resources for replication of more viruses. One of the key components used by the virus for replication is the nucleic acid bases that are needed to produce more viral RNA. Once viral replication begins using the enzyme that the virus has brought in with it, along with host resources, many copies of the viral RNA are made. Required viral proteins are then made; the virus is assembled and packaged.

During this process the virus inhibits host cell functions. This serves the dual purpose of allowing the virus to commandeer the host machinery for its own purposes as well as to ensure that the host cell will die and release all the newly formed viral particles. The newly released viral particles are then free to infect additional cells. What happens if the viral particles are not released? The virus remains intracellular rather than completing the normal viral life cycle, and the result would be a chronic viral infection inside host cells.

It may be that the lack of normal flora in the gut, as well as already elevated levels of the inflammatory mediator TNF, methylation cycle mutations, heavy metal toxicity, and depletion of glutathione due to streptococcal infection set up a predisposing condition for problems with certain vaccines leading to a chronic viral infection. To further exacerbate the condition, it has been found that the tetanus toxin (from the DPT vaccine) can cause the lining of the intestinal tract to peel, leading to diarrhea as well as creating a lack of normal flora. In addition, tetanus toxin inhibits the release of GABA as a result of its action on synaptobrevin. (Vaccines are made by treating the toxins with heat or chemicals, such as formalin, which should denature the toxins). The subsequent vaccination of children with these predisposing conditions, with a live virus such as the MMR vaccine, may allow an otherwise attenuated and non- virulent strain to create an infectious situation by populating the gut. The gut would normally be protected by normal flora and sulfated NAC-glu molecules so that this would not occur. However, given the predisposing conditions, one could end up with the chronic measles infection that has been described by Dr. Andrew Wakefield, and the gut problems addressed by Dr. Jeffrey Bradstreet and Dr. Jerry Kartzinel. In addition to the measles infection, we believe that there are potential problems with chronic viral infections from each of the other viruses in the MMR -- mumps and rubella.

Retroviruses like measles or mumps also have the ability to copy their viral RNA into DNA. This DNA copy of the viral RNA is then stably inserted into the host DNA. As already mentioned, rubella differs from the other two vaccine viruses in that it is a positive stranded RNA virus. However, in the presence of retroviruses, variants of the rubella virus have occurred such that the RNA genome of the virus can also be converted into DNA. This DNA can then stably integrate into the DNA of the host cell, analogous to the situation for mumps and measles. The viral genes will be expressed unless the body has adequate methylation to prevent the expression of these inserted viral genes. Due to an underlying methylation cycle mutations, in addition to the other puzzle pieces already discussed, it is unlikely that the body can prevent this chronic viral expression.

In the case of the MMR vaccine, one of the justifications for vaccination has come from the suggestion of associations between viral infection and diabetes. In the case of rubella virus, it has already been shown to be associated with diabetes. Babies infected with the rubella virus in their mother's womb, who are born with congenitally acquired rubella syndrome, often develop Type I diabetes. One study concluded that rubella virus can infect pancreatic islet cells and that the infection can severely reduce levels of secreted insulin. Like rubella, mumps disease has been strongly associated with the development of Type 1 diabetes. Similar to rubella virus, the mumps virus can infect pancreatic islet cells. It has been found that 85% of children with Type I diabetes have antibodies against the enzyme that converts glutamic acid into GABA (the GAD enzyme, or glutamic acid decarboxylase). This would result in elevated levels of glutamate and reduced levels of GABA. If the pancreas is not functioning optimally (lack of vitamin K, and too much glutamate in the pancreas) then the inflammatory mediators will become glycosylated (have sugars linked onto them), which then calls in more inflammatory mediators to the site. Therefore, many of the potential effects of acute viral infection appear to be similar to the observed issues seen in autism, and may be a result of chronic viral infection with measles, mumps and rubella.

In addition to vaccine issues associated with potential chronic viral infection, there is the issue of the preservatives themselves that are used to maintain the stability of injected substances. The preservatives can contain free glutamate as gelatin, which would directly trigger excitotoxin damage. Many children receive the chickenpox vaccine at the same time as their MMR vaccine. Varivax is stabilized with MSG. The Rotavirus vaccine (used approximately 8/98 to 10/99, 1.5 million doses) contained a contraindication for use specifically for individuals with hypersensitivity to MSG. Other preservatives include thimerosal, phenol, and aluminum. In the case of aluminum, it has been shown that the entry of aluminum into the brain is enhanced when it is coupled to glutamate. Aluminum, once in the brain, is able to trigger additional excitotoxin release and damage. As previously mentioned, mercury is also able to exacerbate excitotoxin damage.

Herpes Viruses

DNA based viruses like chicken pox (Varicella-zoster, or herpes zoster) or Human Herpes Virus 6 (HHV6) can cause problems in addition to the potential problems caused by chronic infection with measles, mumps, and rubella viruses. Dr. Michael Goldberg, Dr. Jeff Galpin and Dr. Kendall Stewart have described the involvement of herpes in conjunction with autism, among others. HHV6 has also been implicated in the demyelinating disease of multiple sclerosis. Recently, HHV6 has been found to be directly correlated with seizure activity. Chicken pox is known to cause neurological damage, particularly during pregnancy. Similar to the situation with the MMR, the virus that is used for the Chicken Pox vaccine is a live attenuated virus. It may be that in individuals with the predisposing conditions already discussed, this virus is also able to establish a chronic infection. If this is the case, then cells that harbor the DNA of the varicella zoster virus may also lead to an accumulation of heavy metals. Other herpes viruses, such as HHV6, may be able to establish chronic viral infections in susceptible individuals with similar results. The potential role of herpes, and other DNA based viruses in autism, is an area that is still evolving.

Other Chronic Viral Infections

A number of other viruses have been implicated in neurological inflammation including CMV (cytomegalovirus), EBV (Epstein-Barr virus), and RSV respiratory syncytial virus). It is impossible at this time to rule out a role for other chronic viral infections in autism. If virus contributes to the pathology of autism by virtue of helping to exacerbate heavy metal retention, then it is possible that any viral infection can be involved. Dr. John Martin of the Center for Complex Infectious Diseases (www.ccid.org) has made us aware of the existence of simian virus 40 (SV40) in early polio vaccines. This is seen in an article in the July issue of New Scientist that reports Soviet oral polio vaccines from the late 1960s found in a freezer at the National Institute for Biological Standards and Controls in the UK were infected with SV40.

Dr. Martin has also conducted additional work with atypical viral infections and believes that they too may be involved in autism. These atypical viruses have been given the name “stealth viruses” as they are able to evade the immune system and lead to chronic infection. These “stealth viruses” appear to have recombined with other genes of cellular, viral or bacterial origin.

Research by Dr. Jean Francois Bach may help to tie together viral infection with yet another piece of the puzzle. Normal individuals harbor autoreactive Tcells that do not attack organs expressing the corresponding autoantigen. For instance, T cells that are specific for myelin basic protein (MBP) or glutamic acid decarboxylase (GAD) can be derived from the peripheral blood of healthy individuals. The research from this group demonstrates that for an autoimmune response to develop, it is not sufficient for T cells to be specific for an autoantigen. The autoreactive cells must also, in addition, be activated. Viral infection has been reported by this group to be sufficient to activate autoreactive T cells.

MHC/HLA Antigens

The MHC (major histocompatibility complex) is a group of genes that code for cell-surface antigens and are the principle determinants of tissue type and transplant compatibility. The HLA antigens are proteins on the surface of human cells that help to identify these cells to the immune system. Differences in HLA antigens are genetically determined.

Dr. Hildreth and his colleagues at Johns Hopkins (Gould et al) believe that the immune response to MHC antigens actually represents the body's original way of defending against retroviruses. They theorize that in the case of HIV, newly formed viruses should bear the HLA proteins from the people they are infecting at the time. If the virus then moves into a second person with dissimilar HLAs, the second person should mount an immune response to the virus.

Several of the live viruses used in vaccines are produced in either human female diploid cells (WI38) or human male diploid cells (MRC5). As the virus is grown and buds through the host cell membrane it picks up host cell components as described above. These components will include HLA antigens or sex specific surface antigens. Individuals with different HLA types may have varying immune responses to these injected HLA antigens as part of the live virus vaccine. Differences in antigenic responses to sex specific cell surface antigens may also be involved in immune responses. Looking at the HLA type of the cell lines used to make live virus vaccines might be worthwhile with an eye toward prescreening for susceptibility to autism.

Differences in susceptibility to measles vaccination have been found to be influenced by the HLA type of an individual. Similarly, HLA antigenic differences are noted for celiac disease, diabetes as well as a number of other autoimmune and inflammatory conditions. Dr. Maddie Hornig has presented results from an animal model that indicate MHC antigens play a role in determining thimerosal related neurotoxicity. HLA type is another area that will likely continue to show a role in autism in the future. It may be that individuals of particular HLA types are more susceptible to predisposing factors involved in this complex condition, similar to the male prevalence in autism that has been noted in the past.

COMT Allelic Variation

As is the case for MTHFr, the COMT enzyme (catechol-O-methyltransferase) has several genetic variants. COMT is also involved in methylation. It is responsible for inactivating several of the neurotransmitters (dopamine, norepinephrine) through the process of transferring methyl groups. The different variant forms of COMT have differing levels of enzyme activity. Individuals with the low activity form of the enzyme would have higher levels of dopamine. Individuals with the high activity enzyme would be more likely to have lower levels of dopamine. In this complex puzzle of autism, dopamine is involved in methylation, therefore the levels of dopamine as a result of the COMT enzyme activity would reflect back on the methylation pathway.

COMT is also responsible for the inactivation of norepinephrine. Differences in norepinephrine and acetylcholine levels may be reflected in terms of the response to new situations. Dr. Yu and Dr. Dayan report that high levels of acetylcholine are associated with the ability to deal with expected uncertainty, while high levels of norepinephrine are required for unexpected uncertainty, as when the aspects of a task are unpredictably changed. Consequently, variations in norepinephrine levels may be a factor in the requirement for "sameness" by so many autistic children. The different allelic variations in COMT activity have also been associated with differential sensitivity to pain; the high activity form of the enzyme was related to better tolerance to pain. The low activity form of the enzyme resulted in greater pain sensitivity. The high activity form of COMT has also been implicated in schizophrenia. Conversely, the low activity form of the enzyme has been associated with rapid cycling bipolar disorder.

Estrogen may help to decrease COMT activity. The antioxidant quercetin is a good substrate for COMT and may also reduce its activity. The exact relationship between the COMT "mutations" and autism is still under investigation. It may be that the different forms of COMT are related to autistic children who are over, or under-methylators. The use of the "blink test" (average number of blinks/minute is between 15-30) may be helpful in the regulation of dopamine. The blink rate varies with the amount of dopamine; less dopamine means fewer blinks.

Muscarinic Receptors/Acetylcholine

Acetylcholine is a neurotransmitter that acts on two types of receptors, nicotinic and muscarinic receptors. Nicotinic receptors are involved with sympathetic nervous system stimulation, while muscarinic receptors are involved with parasympathetic stimulation. The balance between these receptor activities is involved in the sympathetic and parasympathetic imbalances that have been noted in autism. There have been mixed reports when it comes to supplementation of choline to enhance acetylcholine levels in autistic children. Some children appear to respond quite well to choline, while others have negative reactions. Choline supplementation can be particularly dangerous in children with seizures, as choline and acetylcholine have been reported to increase seizure activity. Some children have subclinical seizure activity that has yet to be diagnosed or treated; it can be especially difficult to make the correct judgment with respect to choline supplementation in this specific group of children. (To add to the complexity, vagus stimulation decreases seizure activity in drug resistant epilepsy; vagus nerve stimulation should cause the release of acetylcholine.)

It is important to consider all of the components of any supplement that you give to your children, as they may contain hidden sources of choline or other ingredients that may be a problem. Many transdermal delivery systems (topical delivery gels) contain lecithin as part of the delivery matrix. Lecithin is a source for choline. In addition soy lecithin in topical gel preparations may be a problem for individuals who are allergic to soy.

"Supplementary lecithin requires a special note of caution. Many people take lecithin either under a physician's guidance or from the vitamin counter to eliminate fats and cholesterol from the body. Lecithin is a natural substance that occurs in some plants and animal tissues and in egg yolks. One of its components, choline, is suspect for people with seizures. In a 1983 study, a choline-supplemented diet significantly increased seizures. The researchers concluded, "Our results suggest that supplementation of dietary choline above NORMAL levels might result in increased susceptibility to epileptic seizures. This could result from either a reduced threshold for seizure or from an increase in the rate of seizure development." This conclusion definitely suggests supplementary lecithin with its choline component is not the treatment of choice for people with seizures. (Taken from Epilepsy: A New Approach by Adrienne Richard and Joel Reiter, M.D., Walker and Company, New York, 1995)"

Excess levels of acetylcholine are regulated by the enzyme acetylcholinesterase, which causes the breakdown of acetylcholine. Although it is counter intuitive, a lack of acetylcholinesterase will result in a down-regulation of muscarinic receptors. Potentially this would have the unexpected outcome of <u>high</u> levels of acetylcholine, however with <u>low</u> levels of muscarinic (parasympathetic) receptors. It has been assumed that there is a lack of choline in autism. However, it may instead be a lack of acetylcholine muscarinic receptors. Muscarinic receptors are implicated in processing of cognitive functions, memory, problem solving, regulating pancreatic secretions as well as depressing glutamate release in both the prefrontal cortex and the temporal lobe.

A number of parents believe that their children began the "downward" slide following one or more of the DPT (diphtheria tetanus pertussis) vaccinations. As already mentioned, tetanus toxin (by its action on synaptobrevin) blocks the release of GABA and glycine. In addition tetanus toxin can also inhibit the release of norepinephrine, enkephalins, acetylcholinesterase, and acetylcholine. Tetanus toxin affects the hypothalamus, decreases hormone levels (such as testosterone), causes excessive sympathetic discharge with urinary excretion of catecholamines (i.e. dopamine) and can cause chronic seizure activity. Antibodies against the GAD enzyme (the enzymes that converts glutamate to GABA) have been reported in some cases of tetanus toxicity. Tetanus toxin binds irreversibly. Nerve function can only be returned by the growth of new terminals and synapses.

Toxoid vaccines are made by treating the toxins with heat or chemicals, such as formalin or formaldehyde. The rationale behind this inactivation process is that it should destroy the majority of the toxins ability to inhibit and affect neurotransmitters. However, the toxoid should still be able to stimulate the immune system to produce protective antibodies. Once these protective antibodies are made and bind to the toxin, it should eliminate the toxins ability to bind to the receptors on the host cell membrane. If the body is having difficulties with the immune system, it may be unable to mount a proper antibody response to the injected toxoid. In the absence of antibodies this may allow the toxoid to be free to bind to its target and to interrupt the release of neurotransmittors such as gaba, and glycine and to affect the level of acetylcholinesterase. This would have the consequence of creating imbalances in acetylcholine regulation, with the ultimate result of a decreased number of muscarinic receptors.

The quality control of toxoid vaccines is based on immunogencity and safety testing in animals, which are capable of mounting an appropriate immune response. This leaves open the possibility that the toxoid may behave differently in individuals who do not mount an appropriate immune response. Tetanus toxin behaves like a normal antigen in terms of the immune system, and as such it is recognized in a MHC dependent fashion. The carboxy terminal portion of the toxin is both necessary and sufficient for the ability of the toxin to bind. What this means is that if the carboxy terminus of the toxoid has not been sufficiently denatured it will still be able to bind synaptobrevin and have toxic effects.

In vitro (test tube) analysis of binding activity found that:

> "When *toxoid* or crude toxin is used, non-specific *cleavage of synaptobrevin* substrate occurs" (Kegal et al Federal Agency for Sera and Vaccines Germany).

This indicates that the vaccine toxoid can have similar effects to the toxin itself, especially in the absence of an adequate immune response. Therefore, tetanus toxoid may also be able to inhibit neurotransmitter release. Currently *in vitro* (test tube) tests are not used to monitor the efficiency of toxin inactivation by formaldehyde before use in vaccine preparations.

Nystatin has been shown to prevent cleavage of synaptobrevin by tetanus toxin. Nystatin has also been reported to induce liposome fusion, which may in part compensate for a lack of synaptobrevin. Dr. Sidney Baker and others have described the role of yeast infections in autistic children. Nystatin is often used to treat these infections. Many parents comment on the finding that their children do better on nystatin even in the absence of a yeast infection. It is possible that in addition to its action as an antifungal, the nystatin may be acting to aid in the release of neurotransmittors that have been compromised by tetanus toxoid.

Just as there are "over methylators" and "under methylators" with respect to the methylation pathway, there may be children with different levels of acetylcholine or acetylcholine receptors that in part are determined by their reaction to the DPT vaccines. There may also be a genetic component to this complex piece of the puzzle. We have observed that there is an association between autism and the presence of family members with asthma. The condition of asthma itself is associated with elevations in acetylcholine as well as viral infection (the viruses most commonly associated the asthma attacks are RNA viruses). The microcosm of acetylcholine regulation itself is beginning to emerge as its own complex puzzle within the larger puzzle of autism.

We have had preliminary success in utilizing supplements to enhance muscarinic receptor activity; use of acetyl-L-carnitine, MSM, ashwagandha and ginkgo may be helpful for this purpose. The use of nystatin may also be helpful. In addition, the amino acid alanine has been reported to reverse the inhibitory effects of phenylalanine on acetylcholinesterase activity. It is not known if the use of alanine would help to reverse effects of toxoid inactivation of acetylcholinesterase activity, <u>if</u> that is indeed occurring.

This area is still evolving and is not fully resolved at this time. However, it is important to consider imbalances and irregularities in this system in any treatment plan.

Putting the Pieces Back Together

Our oldest son, Brendan, was different from birth and was diagnosed with Autism in 1996. Our second son, Kyle, was diagnosed with Autism in 1998 after a period of regression. After a lot of interventions they both were verbal but not communicative and had little interest in each other.

In January of 2003 we found Dr. Yasko and we're filled with hope and optimism, but leery when she would say that "it's a marathon not a sprint" because we wanted solutions yesterday. We were sprinting!

Through the protocol we learned how to control exposure to toxins in their environment and customize each of their supplements. We learned the tools that we needed to heal them. We did not have a magic bullet but we were seeing great strides. We talked about how close we were to the end of the marathon and thinking that this is it, this is how life is going to be for our family. We were lucky to be where we were and for the progress they each had made. We were jogging!

In the spring of 2005 we tweaked the supplements and vitamins according to their genetic mutations; slowly and steadily we made more progress. Still no magic bullet, but closer to the end of the marathon. Brendan and Kyle are now able to make friends, fight over the front seat, have a sense of humor and a personality, make the honor roll, play ice hockey, have conversations, talk about girls, and talk, talk, talk. We dream of them being happy, healthy, and independent. We are enjoying them for who they are and who they will become. We are walking!

Dr. Gordon brought Dr. Amy out of her little place in Maine and made her more accessible to others. With the genetics she finally has all the pieces to the puzzle of autism. I encourage each of you to learn about the protocol and use the resources and tools available to heal your children.

It truly is a marathon! Thank you Dr. Amy for walking with us to the finish line.

Michael & Erin Griffin, Parents of Brendan age 13 & Kyle age 10

General Considerations

"Autism Spectrum Disorder" is a catchall phrase, and children with very different biochemical imbalances are put together in this category. Therefore, while there are some universal generalities, the specific plan of treatment depends on the individual needs of each child. However, there are some guidelines that apply to any neurological supplementation program. First, it is recommended that you <u>work in conjunction with a healthcare practitioner</u> when utilizing a detoxification program. Working with someone who has experience in detoxification will be helpful even if they have not used this particular program before. They will have a good idea of what to expect during detoxification and how to deal with the physical and behavioral changes you might encounter through this process.

The program should begin with a really good general supplement that covers the vitamins and minerals, and is high in antioxidant supplements that will lay the groundwork for the more specialized supplements. Preferably this supplement will not contain iron, as iron can exacerbate neurological inflammation. Iron is also necessary for virulence of many bacteria, including streptococci, so limiting iron is useful in limiting bacterial infection, which could trigger additional inflammation. Kyolic garlic has been shown to be effective against ear infections and may be useful in dealing with Streptococci. Also, because of the inherent problem with zinc/copper ratios in many autistic children, any general supplement you choose should not contain copper. Oxidative stress can have pleotropic effects on the body and on inflammation, as has been described by Dr. Woody McGinnis and others specifically with respect to autism. Consequently, the use of additional individual antioxidants in conjunction with a strong antioxidant general vitamin will help to address the issue of oxidative stress.

A hair mineral test, urine test (available from Doctor's Data in Illinois) or a blood test can be used to ascertain that there is no deficiency of copper since prolonged administration of zinc in the absence of copper theoretically could lead to a potential of copper deficiency. In addition, calcium should be included only in limited amounts, and should always be balanced by magnesium.

It has been necessary to temper our suggestions concerning the use of glutathione and sulfur donors since the first edition of this book. Since that time Dr. Yasko has described the impact of CBS mutations that increase the activity of that enzyme. One of the consequences of increased CBS activity is the generation of excess sulfur groups. This can create problems with sulfur toxicity. Rather than making the generic statement that all individuals should get more sulfur/glutathione into the system in as many healthy ways as possible, we have now modified that statement to suggest that an evaluation of CBS status should be made before looking at high dose glutathione supplementation. Glutathione can be well absorbed transdermally and sublingually. There are also a number of sources that have specially formulated glutathione for oral delivery. Glutathione is also delivered via an IV push as well as through the use of a nebulizer. Caution should be used with these later two forms of delivery. We are personally aware of several children who have shown sensitivity to glutathione. Systemic administration or administration directly to the lungs can be extremely dangerous if a child has an anaphylactic reaction to glutathione. Reduced glutathione is reportedly the more potent form of glutathione; NADH can be used as a supplement to help recycle reduced glutathione. The use of NADH is especially important for those using glutathione via an IV push. If NADH is not supplemented then the body may "steal" NADH from other internal pathways in an attempt to recycle the glutathione. We have seen cases where children became depleted in NADH after the use of IV glutathione without supplementation with NADH. In these cases the Krebs cycle may become compromised.

There are also a number of supplements that will indirectly boost glutathione levels, these include: milk thistle, alpha lipoic acid, N-acetyl-cysteine/vitamin C, MSM, aloe and rosemary among others. While glutamate (or glutamic acid or glutamine) and cysteine are precursors in the formation of glutathione, they are also excitotoxins and will trigger more inflammation in the brain; therefore it is best not to use those items directly as supplements to boost glutathione levels. Foods/supplements that are naturally high in sulfur include garlic, broccoli, onions, and foods high in quercetin. The level of cysteine in the transsulfuration pathway determines if taurine or glutathione is produced via this route. The pathway is shunted in the direction of taurine production rather than glutathione production under conditions of high level cysteine. The use of low doses of curcumin is often helpful in shifting the synthesis to glutathione rather than taurine.

If the liver is healthy it can make sufficient glutathione -- one of the most important antioxidants in the body. The liver is also critical as the site of detoxification of waste products for the body. Anything that makes the liver healthier will help; this would include some of the supplements already mentioned such as milk thistle, carnitine, NAC, dandelion (also high in vitamin A), as well as SAMe and B vitamins. The use of depakane (valproic acid) can deplete carnitine. Children who are taking valproic acid to reduce seizure activity should consider supplementation with carnitine.

In individuals where chronic yeast or fungal infection is evident, it is important to restore the normal functioning of the intestinal tract. Supplement with a really good source of vitamin K, agents to limit yeast formation (which occurs as a result of lack of normal flora) and digestive enzymes. Supplements that will help with digestion and yeast overgrowth include lactoferrin, digestive enzymes, and probiotics.

Individuals should consider supplements to help to detoxify the excess glutamate in the system. These would include branched chain amino acids (mixture of leucine, isoleucine and valine only), pycnogenol, and grape seed extract. Magnesium is critical as it regulates the excess calcium from flowing into the nerves and killing them. Epsom salt baths (magnesium sulfate) are useful particularly if the bathing water is high in chloride and fluoride. Chloride blocks the action of sulfur in the body. Limited amounts of zinc and calcium are fine, but too much will increase nerve damage.

Supplements that add energy (oxygen and ATP) to the brain will help it to detoxify the inflammatory reactions caused by excess glutamate and heavy metals, which trigger glutamate release. These supplements include ginkgo, vinpocetine, NADH, CoQ10, ribose, and carnitine. It is important to use NADH with glutathione to maintain the glutathione in a reduced state. Carnitine actually helps to increase the energy in the mitochondria, which are the energy producing organelles inside each cell. Carnitine is also useful in repairing liver damage. Acetyl L carnitine is another form of carnitine that is particularly useful for helping to balance the parasympathetic aspect of the nervous system as it has been reported to increase muscarinic receptors. Ginkgo is also described to increase muscarinic receptor density. Ribose has been documented to raise ATP levels. Elevated levels of ATP will in turn help to generate energy to aid in the removal of glutamate from the brain.

B vitamins are crucial for nerve health. They also help to form the sulfur containing amino acids. A really good B complex is important. In addition, B12 can be taken sublingually so that it is not degraded in the stomach. B12 helps with energy as well as repairs nerves. B12 is also important in helping to compensate for the MTHFr mutation that seems to be present in most of these children. It is important to take B vitamins as a complex, as it has been shown that taking a single B vitamin will deplete the levels of the other B vitamins and this occurs in a dose dependent fashion. For example, a central inflammatory mediator in other neurological inflammation is homocysteine. Lack of particular B's will increase the homocysteine levels in the blood. In the case of B vitamins a little bit of each of the specific B's with higher levels of particular B's has given the best results.

High levels of B6 or P5P can sometimes cause a child to become more "stimmy". In addition to its role in helping to convert glutamate to GABA, B6 is involved in a number of other enzymatic reactions in the body. For example, B6 helps in the metabolism of tryptophan, in its breakdown to nicotinamide. Several intermediates in this pathway, Kynurenic acid and Quinolinic acid, are involved in regulating glutamate and excitotoxins. Kynurenic acid helps to protect against excitotoxins. Quinolinic acid stimulates the glutamate receptors and can lead to excitotoxin damage. Vitamin B6 helps to convert Kynurenine to Quinolinic acid, and may therefore lead to increased levels of the excitotoxin Quinolinic acid. In children with high levels of glutamate it might therefore be wise to use small amounts of B6 and P5P. Similarly by virtue of its structure, folate contains glutamate. Again, it may be prudent to use small amounts of several derivatives of folate rather than large amounts of a single source of folate. B6 and P5P also help to push the CBS reaction as well as to aid in the conversion of kynurenic to quinolinic. This would suggest that only low levels of P5P should be utilized for individuals with chronic bacterial issues and CBS up regulations.

Another basic supplementation issue to consider is increasing the intake of Omega 3 oils (essential fatty acids like EPA and DHA) while restricting the intake of Omega 6 oils. The proper ratio of essential fats is essential for the development of healthy neurons. An imbalance exists today in virtually every one of us; Americans have a marked excess of Omega 6 oils such as soy and corn oil with a major deficiency of healthy Omega 3 oils from flax and fish. This imbalance of fatty acids increases inflammation and thus contributes to ill health. The proper levels of Omega 3 fatty acids are able to reduce the levels of inflammatory mediators including cox2, IL1 and TNF alpha. Insufficient levels of Omega 3 have been linked to everything from cancer and heart disease to our current epidemic of neurological diseases. The role of omega 3 fatty acids, in autism in particular, has been described by Dr. Andrew Stoll and others.

A healthy ratio is now believed to be 2:1 of omega 6 oils over Omega 3 in our diet. (There are some who prefer a 5:2 ratio). Researchers find that today most of us are getting a 20 fold (or greater) excess of Omega 6 over Omega 3 oils in our diet. Dr. Garry Gordon and Dr. Herb Joiner-Bey have written a book on this subject "The Omega-3 Miracle" that describes the extensive research on this vital nutrient including dramatic successes in dealing with various mental illnesses including Manic Depression and ADD. However, individuals with increased CBS enzyme activity as well as those with particular MTHFR mutations (A1298C) may also have special issues with lipids and may benefit from lower overall doses of fatty acids. We also would limit the intake of high glycemic foods, and limit the intake of all processed foods with their heavy load of chemicals, preservatives, pesticides etc. In order to balance our Omega 3 intake, we have to lower our excessive intake of Omega 6 oils. We also need to eliminate high fructose corn syrup, which we now find everywhere, even in crackers.

Another general area to address is water. Many parents are concerned about metals or chemicals in their water supply. This is a valid concern as it is important to look at the total body burden of toxic metals and chemicals. Special bottled waters are available, however, they are often quite costly. Drinking a few bottles of "special water" daily and fulfilling the rest of the days needs with distilled water or with water purified by reverse osmosis can reach a reasonable balance. While there is no perfect solution to the water issue, if the child is supplementing with a low dose of a safe chelating agent and bathing in a chelating agent this will help to reduce toxin buildup over time. There are a wide variety of bottled waters; our personal favorites are Penta water (to increase oxygenation) and Nariwa water (for the enhanced value of magnetism on the nerves).

One place where individuals can have difficulties with a supplement plan is the source/quality of the supplements and vitamins they are using. We have all heard people say "Oh, I've tried that before, it doesn't work", only to find that when they use a high quality version of that same supplement, it does in fact make a difference for them. Alternatively, there are cases where individuals were following these suggested protocols with great success, only to find that they were not doing as well when they switched to another brand of supplement, or one that was not stored properly. It is therefore important to consider "supplement quality" as an aspect of any nutritional plan. Supplements are not regulated. As a result supplement quality can vary greatly. Also, supplements can go off or spoil (similar to fresh produce) if they are not stored or shipped properly. Consequently, it is not simply a matter of supplement brand, it is also important to consider other factors, such as how it was stored (in a hot stockroom), how long it's been sitting on the shelf and how it was shipped.

Those of us practicing alternative health care did not set out with the intention of selling supplements. However, we have found that not all supplements are made under the same high standards that are necessary to have successful results. Over time we have found that it is important for you to use the proper tools to take charge of your health. One of these tools includes the use of supplements. Use good judgment in choosing your source of supplements. Please do not be guided simply by the price. The difference of a few dollars may mean the difference between a successful supplement program and one that is mediocre. (Information on specific supplements that have been "hand picked" by Dr. Amy is available from www.holisticheal.com, www.longevityplus.com, www.longevityplus-rna.com, www.antiageing-nutrition.com and www.holistichealth.com).

Step 1: Program for Neurological Inflammation

The first step in the Program for Neurological Inflammation is removing excitotoxin triggers from the diet. This simply involves reading labels and closely monitoring food and supplement intake to avoid excitotoxins. In addition, it is important to limit the intake of calcium to prevent damage to neurons. Excess excitotoxins cause an imbalance in the flow of calcium, which leads to activation of a complex inflammatory cascade, release of inflammatory mediators and ultimately the death of neurons. Dr. Mark Neveu, President of NFAM (National Foundation of Alternative Medicine) has a wonderful and vitally important way of describing the relationship between glutamate and calcium in creating excitotoxin damage. He views glutamate as the gun, and calcium as the bullet. If both glutamate (and other excitotoxins) and calcium are kept under control, it is possible to limit the excitotoxin damage.

Most autistic children already follow a restricted diet - limiting the intake of gluten and casein. In addition, we recommend avoiding any sources of glutamate (and other excitotoxins) as well as keeping calcium under control. By adding these other dietary parameters, it is possible to limit further excitotoxin damage to the body. Calcium is kept to a minimum in the early stages of our program by limiting its ingestion and with the supplementation of magnesium and zinc. The back of this book lists various names of excitotoxins so that they can be avoided in the diet. It is also important to understand that high protein means more excitotoxins.

We recognize that the complete list of foods with excitotoxins may initially seem overwhelming. It is fortunately not necessary to eliminate <u>every</u> molecule, but it is necessary to limit what we find has been the excessive intake that contributes to the overall load of glutamate and related excitotoxins. It is important to stop the inflammatory process created by these excitotoxin triggers. Halting this inflammatory cascade is achieved with a number of supplements as well as RNA-based formulas that are designed to mitigate the inflammatory process. We have found that these RNA formulas make a tremendous difference in helping to turn the tide of inflammation that even the best supplement protocols will not handle on their own.

Since one area of concern in autism is on lowering inflammation, it may be interesting to review a book by Richard Fleming MD, "Stop Inflammation Now". Although it is focused on heart disease, it, nonetheless, provides useful up to date thinking about the benefits from dramatic dietary changes along the lines of what you will be following for your child. There are still minor disagreements that your authors have with this book as well as others along the same vein, but it is useful for background reading to learn that it is increasingly clear that the American diet has set the stage for a variety of inflammatory disorders.

It is important to understand that the body is both efficient and conservative with mediators when it comes to inflammation. The very same inflammatory mediators that cause inflammation surrounding the nerves or in the gut in autism are also the culprits for the inflammation we see in heart disease, arthritis and even certain cancers.

Finally, during this first phase, it is necessary to support impaired systems and to lay the groundwork to repair and generate new neurons. This is accomplished with a variety of herbs, vitamins, and nutritional supplements that serve as antioxidants and help to reinforce the child's diet. The idea is to compensate for any imbalances in the body due to the malfunctioning of a number of organ and metabolic systems, many of which have been previously described by Dr. Jon Pangborn. The number of supplements utilized varies from approximately 5 to 50 or more, depending on the severity and the number of the imbalances in an individual child. The systems or imbalances that may require supplementation include the pancreas, the intestinal tract, excessive acid production in the stomach, the liver, hormonal imbalances, thyroid, adrenals, and neurotransmitter imbalances among others. This may seem like a lot of supplements, and in some cases it is. However, the ultimate goal is the reversal of accumulated damage. Nerve damage is a process; by the time an individual recognizes that they have neurological problems, more than 50% of their neurons may have been damaged causing obvious neurological symptoms. It takes time and commitment in order to halt and reverse this process. How long does it take to grow a new neuron? No one really knows. For years it was widely believed that it did not happen at all, but we now know that it does happen. What we do know is that when we have an individual who commits to their program and stays with it, together we are able to achieve incredible results. Remember, this is a marathon, not a sprint.

The suggested supplementation protocol is broken into categories. It is not necessary to take every supplement in every category. However, depending upon the severity of an individual case of autism, you may find it necessary to use every supplement listed. It is always possible that a particular child may be sensitive to an individual herb or supplement. It is best for this reason to add supplements slowly to the program, allowing several days to be certain that the newly added supplements agree with the child before progressing to add additional new supplements. Yes, it will take a while to introduce all the new supplements. It is important to remember to be calm and patient, and not feel rushed to get through the program.

An alternative to slowly adding supplements and allowing several days to determine a child's reaction to a particular supplement is to take advantage of energy testing. There are a number of qualified individuals who will provide energy testing for you and your child to determine which are the most appropriate supplements for your child's individual program. There are also a number of reputable sources for EAV equipment for home or office use that will aid in supplement choices based on an individual child's particular needs. Many EAV practitioners also practice homeopathy. The use of homeopathy for autism works well in conjunction with the protocol we have described. Our protocol has not been found to interfere with the use of homeopathic drugs, and the use of homeopathics may have a synergistic effect with this program.

The suggested dosage on any supplement listed in our protocol is 1/2 to 1 capsule or tablet unless otherwise noted. This will be well below the dosage suggested on the labels of the bottles. The approach is to try to re-balance a number of pathways in the body simultaneously. If you begin to think about the body as a roadway system, imagine that you are supplementing the main road, the side roads, and the back roads all at the same time. This requires a small amount of a large number of supplements. This is the way the body is accustomed to working, having multiple pathways and feedback systems to get to the same point.

Overview of Entire Program - Steps 1, 2, & 3

1) Begin by ordering a test to look at imbalances in the methylation cycle (www.testing4health.com). A nutrigenomic profile will help you to evaluate the relative contribution of any underlying genetic susceptibility to autism. A specific knowledge of where the methylation cycle mutations reside will help you to make decisions concerning nutritional support to bypass these mutations. While you are waiting for your nutrigenomic test results begin with Step 1 support (described below). This includes organ support as well as a heavy concentration on balancing glutamate and GABA in the body.

2) Once the organ systems are well supported and glutamate and GABA are more in balance you can look at supporting the body to address chronic bacterial issues which can also lead to aluminum excretion. Support includes the use of CCK/BioThyro, along with low dose EDTA, Beyond Clean in the bath, malic acid, horsetail grass and the rest of the gut program as needed. (Rotating normal flora, rotating gut herbs, Microbial support and Mycology Support formulas, IMF 5, IMF 7, and Candex). It is useful to run spot urine toxic metal tests at this time to monitor the excretion of aluminum that accompanies bacterial detoxification.

3) If you still have not received your nutrigenomic profile, then consider the use of Metals formulas in conjunction with your doctor and the use of the viral support herbs described in Step 2. You can also look at adding in the Methylation Support RNA formula at this time along with Moducare and elderberry if you are going to support the body in a general way to address chronic viral issues. Frequent urine tests for toxic heavy metals and essential minerals are critical at this point.

4) Once you receive your nutrigenomic profile begin by supporting CBS up regulations and addressing ammonia. If there are no CBS up regulations you can go on to the next step. If you are addressing CBS up regulations, wait about a month before progressing to the next step.

5) Next, move to more comprehensive methylation cycle support including 1/4 Folapro, 1/4 Intrinsic B12, additional B12, SAMe (depending on COMT/VDR status), 1/4 nucleotides, HHC general vitamin, mixture of PS/PC/PE (or Pedi Active depending on COMT/VDR status), and Methylation Support formula (if not yet added). If you have not started to monitor urine for toxic metals and essential minerals, this is the point to begin, as supporting the methylation pathway will trigger detoxification.

6) It may take months for the detoxification of metals to abate and for the methylation cycle to get back in balance. Once methionine, FIGLU and methylmalonic acid levels are in normal range, you can consider decreasing the use of PS/PC/PE and/or PediActive to once daily and stopping the use of any additional TMG (beyond what is in the HHC general). You can look at adding in DMG to shift the focus of the methylation cycle toward the MTR/MTRR pathway rather than the BHMT enzyme.

7) Support for BH4 deserves special consideration. BH4, or tetrahydrobiopterin is needed for neurotransmitter synthesis, detoxification of ammonia, lipid processing and appears to play

a critical role in language development along with GABA and dopamine. We can think of BH4 as a stool with three legs. One leg can be labeled “CBS up regulations”. The second leg can be labeled “MTHFR A1298C” and the third leg can be labeled “chronic bacteria/aluminum”. In order to have a stable stool, or stable BH4 levels it requires that all three legs be sturdy. If there are CBS up regulations it weakens one of the legs of the stool. The more total CBS up regulations the weaker that particular leg is. If there are MTHFR A1298C mutations this impairs a second leg of the stool. Chronic bacterial infection which can lead to retention of aluminum causes issues with the third leg of the stool.

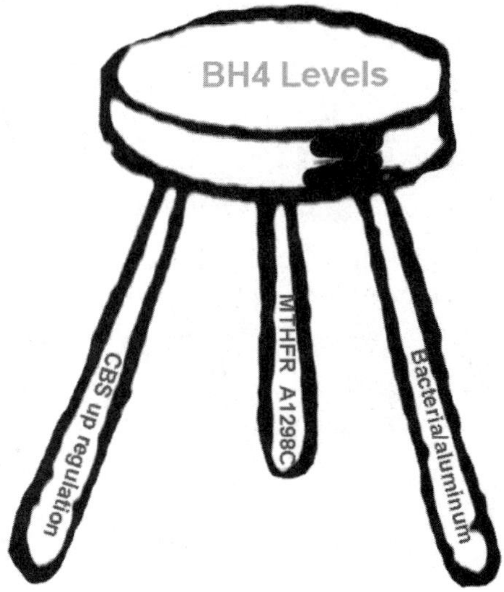

Aluminum inhibits the enzyme that is needed to synthesize BH4. Between aluminum (due to bacterial infection) which inhibits the ability to make BH4, the A1298C mutation which disrupts the ability to recycle and regenerate BH4 and the CBS up regulations which use up BH4 faster than it can be supplied, individuals who are CBS +, MTHFR A1298C + and have chronic bacterial and aluminum issues may be severely depleted in BH4. It is important to address all three legs of the BH4 stool by supporting the body to address chronic bacteria/aluminum, supporting the MTHFR A1298C mutation and addressing CBS/ammonia issues.

Step 1: Suggested Protocol for Neurological Inflammation

Vitamins/ Minerals/ Antioxidants to Lay the Nutritional Groundwork:

- Complete Vitamin & Ultra Antioxidant
- Vitamin D
- Vitamin C
- Cell Food/ BioNativus Multimins
- Vitamin E +mixed tocopherols
- Liquid Selenium drops
- Liquid Molybdenum drops
- Liquid Manganese drops
- Iodine (depending on levels)
- Nerve Calm RNA Formula (2X/day or as needed)
- Health Foundation RNA Formula (2X/day or as needed)
- Stress RNA Formula (2X/day or as needed)
- Behavior RNA Formula (2X/day or as needed)
- Bowel RNA Formula (2X/day or as needed)
- Stomach pH RNA Formula (2X/day or as needed)

Support Liver Health/ Increase Glutathione/ Increase Sulfur:
*(Use **LIMITED** sulfur support if you suspect a CBS up regulation)*

- Milk thistle
- B complex/SAMe (depending on nutrigenomics for COMT and CBS)
- Alpha lipoic acid (only 1/2 should be fine regardless of CBS status)
- Taurine (depending on levels on urine AA test)
- Broccoli
- Rosemary
- Garlic
- Sublingual Glutathione
- Oral GSH Glutathione (some parents prefer IV glutathione)
- Glucosamine/MSM
- Chondroitin Sulfate
- Dandelion root
- Carnitine

Cod Liver Oil
Ora-Liv
Organ Support RNA
Shark oil
N-acetyl cysteine w/ Quercetin
Vitamin C with Rose Hips (500mg c for every 250 mg NAC)
Creams:
Glutathione cream
Magnesium sulfate cream
Alpha lipoic acid cream
Glucosamine/ MSM cream

Support for Kidney Health:
SAMe
Dandelion Leaf
Kidney Support RNA
Cranberry
Curbita

Supplements to Aid in Protection from Excess Calcium:
Magnesium
Vinpocetine
Zinc (25-40mg/day)

Support to Increase Calcium:
Nettle
Chamomille
Chervil
HHC cal/mag/vit D/vit K

Supplements to Aid in the Balance of Glutamate and GABA:
Branched Chain Amino Acids (ONLY leu/ileu/val)
(discontinue immediately if urine smells like “maple syrup”)
Pycnogenol
Grape seed extract
GABA

- Sublingual GABA Calm/ Glycine
- Sublingual methylcobalamin (B12)
- Sublingual cyanocobalamine (B12)
- Sublingual hydroxycobalamin (B12)
- ZEN
- L-Theanine
- Taurine (depending on urine AA test levels)
- Cats Claw
- Trehalose
- Nerve Calm RNA
- Lithium orotate (depending on levels on urine essential test)
- Liposomal B12
- Progesterone cream
- Valerian root

Supplements to Support the Pancreas:

- Ora-Pancreas
- Vitamin K
- Super Digestive Enzymes
- Ayur-Gymnema
- Apex Lean (CCK)
- CCK Support RNA
- Pig duodenum
- ProLongevity RNA

Decrease Bacteria/ Repopulate GI Tract:

- Rotate probiotics (one each day of the week):
  - UltraDairy enzymes
  - Kyodophilus
  - Prescript assist
  - Suprema dophilus
  - Toueff
  - Allerdophilus
  - Colon Health Support
  - Florastor
- Rotate Antimicrobial Herbs (choice based on CDSA

sensitivity tests):

- Oregon grape
- Myrrh
- Neem
- Goldenseal
- Uva Ursi (limited use)
- Cranberry
- Oregamax
- Caprylic acid
- Barberry
- Olive extract

Additional Microbial Support:

- CCK
- BioThyro
- CCK Support RNA
- Microbial Support RNA
- Stomach pH RNA
- Bowel Support RNA
- IMF 5
- Lactoferrin
- Grapefruit seed extract
- ARA 6

Chelate Aluminum Released by Microbes:

- EDTA
- Malic acid
- Horsetail grass

Support to Balance/ Repopulate GI Tract/ Decrease Yeast:

- Rotate probiotics (one each day of the week):
    - UtraDairy enzymes
    - Kyodophilus
    - Prescript assist
    - Suprema dophilus
    - Toueff

Allerdophilus
Colon Health Support

Additional Supplements for Yeast Support:
- Candex
- IMF 7
- Lactoferrin
- Oregamax
- Uva ursi
- Caprylic acid
- CCK
- BioThyro
- Stomach pH RNA
- CCK Support RNA
- Mycology Support RNA
- Buffer pH supplement

Support to Balance Parasites:
- Paradex

Support to Reducing Stims:
- Nettle
- Behavior RNA Formula (as needed)
- Stress RNA Formula (as needed)
- Inositol or IP6

Support Membrane Fluidity:
- Phosphatidyl serine or Pedia-active chewable
- Essential Fatty Acid Mixture
- Neuromins (DHA)
- Policosanol

Support for the Immune System/ Thymus/ Spleen:
- Colostrum
- IVIG
- Ora -triplex

- Immuno-forte
- Peptizyde (1/4 to 1/2 daily for immune support) or
- Serenaide (1/4 to 1/2 daily for immune support)
- Spirulina
- IP6
- Mycoceutics mushroom w/ beta glucan
- Kidney Support RNA
- Transfer Factor

Aid in Helping Inflammation Around Nerves:

- Health Foundation RNA (as needed)
- HyperImmune RNA (limited amounts for COMT V158M+)
- Behavior Support RNA
- Nettle
- Skull cap
- Boswellia
- Curcumin (limited amounts for COMT V158M+)
- Skull cap
- Chamomile
- Quercetin
- Petadolex (Butterbur)
- Cherry Fruit Extract
- Advanced Joint Support RNA
- Stress RNA
- Lung Support RNA
- Colostrum
- Kidney Support RNA

Supplements to Support Mitochondrial/ Krebs Energy:

- CoQ 10
- NADH
- Ginkgo Biloba
- Oxydrene
- Idebenone
- ATP
- Vinpocetine

L-Carnitine
Melatonin
Krebs zinc
Krebs magnesium/potassium chelate
Riboflavin
Pantothenic acid (if levels of pantothenic acid are low on OAT/MAT)
Carntine fumarate (if fumarate levels are low on OAT/MAT)
Vitamin E succinate (if succinate levels are low on OAT/MAT)
Malic acid (if malate levels are low on OAT/MAT)
Magnesium citrate (if citrate levels are low on OAT/MAT)
Pyruvate (if pyruvate levels are low on OAT/MAT)

Support Balance Zinc/ Copper:
Carnosine
Rosemary
EDTA (just 1X/day at this stage)
Molybdenum
E lyte zinc
Krebs zinc
Chewable zinc with slippery elm
Beyond Clean

Supplements to Support the Gut:
Curcumin
Slippery Elm
Colostrum
Glucosamine/MSM
Mastica Gum
Bowel RNA Formula (as needed)
Slippery Elm
Marshmallow
Colostrum
Masrica gum

Supplements to Aid in Constipation:

- Artichoke
- Yellow Dock
- Cascara Sagrada
- Aloe Vera
- Magnesium
- Cod Liver oil
- Rhubarb

Note: *If supplements are listed in more than one category the intention is to take the supplement only once a day. They are listed in each category to give a sense of the multiple uses of the individual supplements.*

Indications for Step 1 Organ Support

Please Note: *It is NOT necessary to run every lab test mentioned or to use every supplement listed. The purpose of this list is to help you to determine the type of organ support needed for Step 1 of the program based on lab tests that you have already run and have in your files. The DVD entitled Dr. Amy's Supplement Guide is also a useful aid in supplement choice for Step 1.*

Lab Tests Indicating a Need for **Liver Support**:

- Elevated AST (SGOT)
- Elevated ALT (SGPT)
- Elevated alkaline phosphatase (ALP)
- Elevated lactate dehydrogenase (LDH)
- Elevated billirubin
- Elevated cholesterol
- Elevated triglycerides
- Long term chelation with sulfur based chelating agents
- High level excretion of toxic metals on fecal tests

Lab Tests Indicating a Need for **Kidney Support**:

- Elevated BUN
- Urine excretion/detox of metals for prolonged periods

Lab Tests Indicating a Need for **Pancreatic Support**:

- Consistently elevated glucose
- Consistently low glucose
- Elevated triglycerides
- VDR Fok + - or VDR Fok + +
- Imbalances in pancreatic elastase on a CDSA
- Imbalances in chymotrypsin values on a CDSA
- Imbalances in SCFA (Iso-butyrate, iso-valerate and n-valerate) on CDSA
- Imbalances in LCFA on a CDSA

Lab Tests Indicating a Need to **Decrease Calcium**:

- Elevated calcium relative to magnesium on a urine essential element test
- Elevated calcium relative to magnesium on a red blood cell element test
- Stims

Lab Tests Indicating a Need to **Increase Calcium**:

- Calcium below the range of low end normal on a urine essential test
- Calcium below the range of low end normal on a RBC element test
- High level excretion of lead should check urine calcium levels

Lab Tests Indicating a Need for **Glutamate/ GABA Balance**:

- Elevated glutamate, glutamine, glutamic acid on urine AA Test
- Elevated aspartate, aspartic acid on urine AA Test
- Low GABA (gamma aminobutyric acid) on a urine AA Test
- Low GABA on a Neurotransmitter Test

Elevated quinolinic on OAT/Metabolic Test
Seizures
Stims
Poor eye contact
Aggressive behavior

Lab Tests Indicating a Need for **Immune Support**:
Imbalances on ImmunoSciences Test Panels

Lab Tests Indicating a Need to Address **Bacterial Imbalances**:
History of chronic ear infections
Maternal history of Streptococcal infection
History of bacterial pneumonia
Streptococcus, E.coli on CDSA
Other bacterial pathogens on CDSA
Elevated kynurenic on OAT/Metabolic Test, CONFIRM with CDSA
Elevated quinolinic on OAT/Metabolic Test, CONFIRM with CDSA
Low gut pH

Lab Tests Indicating a Need to Address **Yeast Imbalances**:
Elevated arabinose on OAT/Metabolic Test, CONFIRM with CDSA
Presence of yeast on CDSA
Low gut pH, CONFIRM with CDSA

Lab Tests Indicating a Need to Address **Parasites**:
Parasites on a CDSA

Lab Tests Indicating a Need to Address **Helicobacter**:
Helicobacter test

Lab Tests Indicating a Need to Support **Inflammatory Imbalances**:
Elevated chymotrypsin test levels
CRP above normal range on blood work

Elevated IL 6 on blood work
Elevated TNF alpha on blood work
Chronic bacterial infection (see lab list above)
Low gut pH
Allergic Rashes

Lab Tests Indicating a Need to Address **Zinc/ Copper Ratio**:
Elevated copper relative to zinc on a urine essential element test
Elevated copper relative to zinc on blood work
Low levels of ceruloplasmin on blood work
Red hair, CONFIRM with a essential mineral test

Lab Tests Indicating a Need to Address **Glutathione or Low Sulfur Values**:
Low glutathione on tests (for low reduced glutathione (GSH) but high oxidized glutathione (GssG) consider NADH first, then rerun test for reduced glutathione levels)
GST polymorphisms
Low values on a hepatic detox profile
Low sulfur test values

Tests Indicating a Need to Address **Mitochondrial Support/ Krebs Cycle**:
Elevated suberic on OAT/Metabolic analysis test
Low levels of Krebs cycle intermediates

Step 2: Program for Toxin Elimination

The next phase of the protocol helps to remove toxins from the body. This is the "elimination" part of the program. Brooks and his colleagues have demonstrated a strategy to eliminate chronic stores of retrovirus in the body that serve as a source for renewed viral infection. Their work has shown that activating the latently infected cells makes them susceptible to therapy and depletes the bulk of the reservoir of infected cells. Expanding on this philosophy, we have found that it is possible to support the body with supplements that should help to eradicate the latent reservoir of virus. As the virus is eliminated, we see a release of stored metals from the body. Supplements are added during this phase to help eliminate both chronic virus and metals.

Detoxification can be very stressful on the body. It is therefore important to allow sufficient time for Step One before progressing to Step Two. Organ systems should be functioning better, the "stims" should be down, there should be better eye contact, better sleep, and an improvement in the bowels and absorption before progressing to Step Two. The comprehensive supplementation program that was used in Step One should be continued to ensure that the immune system and other organs are well supported during the elimination process. The support program to address chronic bacteria and aluminum excretion can also be used prior to instituting the rest of Step Two. Any new supplements in the Detoxification part of the program should be added in the same way those new supplements were added in Step One. Again, it is not necessary to take every supplement in every category. However, depending upon the severity of the individual you may find it necessary to use every supplement listed. It is always possible that a particular child may be sensitive to an individual herb or supplement. It is best for this reason to add supplements slowly to the program, allowing several days to be certain that the newly added supplements agree with the child before progressing to add additional new supplements. Yes, it will take a while to introduce all the new supplements. Again, this is a marathon, not a sprint! The suggested dosage on any supplement is 1/2 to 1 whole capsule or tablet unless otherwise noted. This will be well below the dosage suggested on the labels of the bottles.

The purpose of Step 2 is to support the body to allow for excretion of toxic metals through the release of chronic viral and bacterial infection in the body (if that has not already been addressed as part of Step 1). This is based on the theory that bacteria help to retain aluminum in the body and that chronic viral infection allows for heavy metal accumulation. This Step begins by looking at the nutrigenomic profile to bypass methylation cycle mutations with the use of supplements (see the book Genetic Bypass for more detailed information on nutrigenomics). Since the methylation cycle is so critical to silencing virus, and supporting the immune system, simply allowing the methylation cycle to function is often enough to allow for viral, bacterial and metal detoxification.

Overview of Step 2

1) Address CBS/ammonia imbalances using the ammonia support program. This is an important first step so that added methylation cycle support does not lead to increased levels of ammonia, hydrogen sulfide and other toxic sulfur byproducts. **If there are no CBS up regulations you can proceed to number 3.**

2) Wait at least one month before looking to add the rest of methylation cycle support as indicated by the nutrigenomic profile. During this time period you can look at integrating the use of the comprehensive gut/bacterial support program while the CBS/ammonia issues get in better balance.

3) Support the rest of the methylation cycle imbalances using support for both pathways around the methylation cycle. You are looking to support the "long way" around the cycle via the MTHFR/MTR/MTRR as well as the "short cut" through the cycle via the BHMT enzyme.

4) Creatinine levels will increase as a function of proper methylation cycle function as well as by virtue of the decreased ammonia levels as CBS up regulations are addressed. Increased creatinine will cause detoxification reactions.

5) Increased beta alanine, anserine, and carnosine may be seen as the "short cut" around the methylation cycle as it is supported and ammonia levels drop.

6) Once the levels of beta alanine, anserine, and carnosine drop you can consider the addition of DMG. This will emphasize the long route around the cycle rather than the short cut.

7) Add in metals RNA program if needed.

The role of the Folapro, intrinsic B12, nucleotides and folinic is to compensate for the methylation cycle mutations. This will open up the pathway, and in doing so will allow the proper expansion of T cells to aid in viral elimination. It is for this precise reason that we ask you to WAIT to add these supplements, until the body has had a chance to rebalance in Step One, and then have the immune support necessary in Step Two before beginning a detoxification process.

There seems to be a tremendous amount of confusion in the literature concerning 5 methyl folate. Only 5 methyl folate will bypass the MTHFr mutation; 5 formyl folate has other advantages, but it will not bypass the mutation. In order to go from 5 formyl THF to 5 methyl THF requires MTHFr. The product called Folapro is clearly 5 methyl THF. There are products on the market labeled as folinic acid that are 5 formyl THF and others labeled folinic that are 5 methyl THF. Given the confusion, it is safer to use a product based on the chemical formula, rather than to use it based on its name on the label.

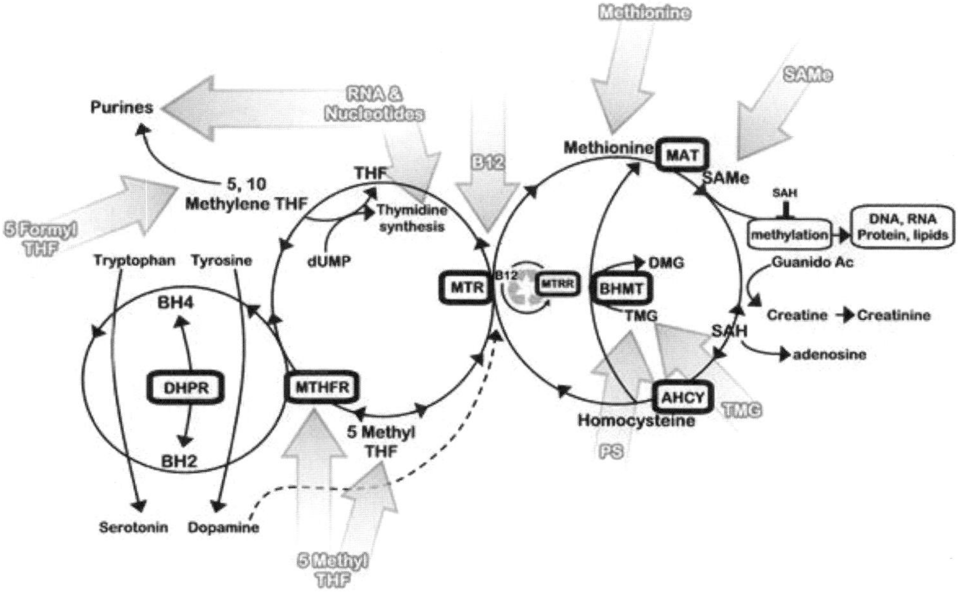

There are two pathways that will take you around the methylation cycle from homocysteine to methionine. The first is the "long way" around the cycle via the MTR and MTRR enzymes that requires B12 and the forward reaction of the MTHFR (where the C677T impairs the activity) for function. The other is a "short cut" through the middle of the cycle that bypasses MTR, MTRR and MTHFR via the BHMT enzyme. If you think of this portion of the cycle as a clock, the BHMT enzyme can use phosphatidyl serine, phosphatidyl choline and TMG as substrates to go directly from homocysteine at 6:00 to methionine at 12:00 skipping 7:00 through 11:00. The use of phosphatidyl choline, phosphatidyl serine and TMG therefore help to bypass these mutations. This backdoor reaction (or short cut) generates more norepinephrine relative to dopamine. The BHMT enzyme is also triggered by stress.

Imbalances in dopamine relative to norepinephrine have been implicated in ADD and ADHD behaviors.

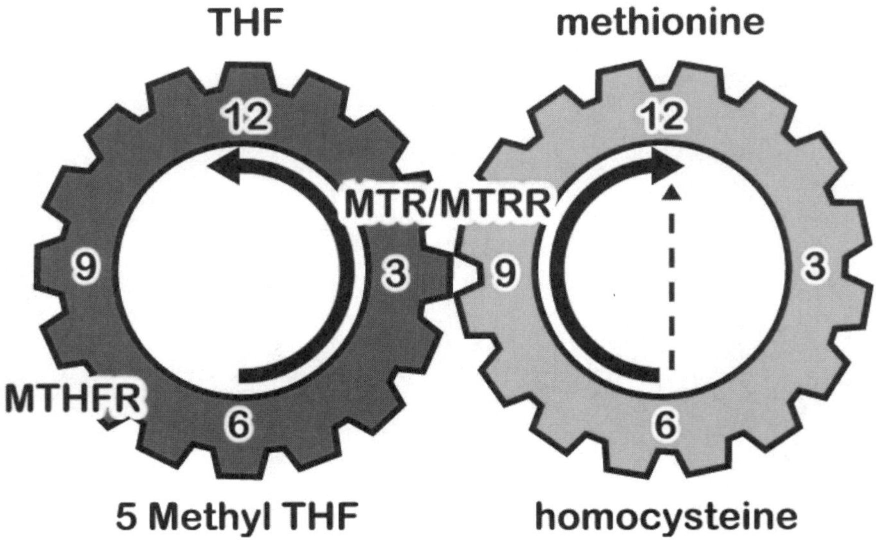

Initially it is simply important to get the methylation cycle moving again for individuals with mutations in these pathways. If the pathway has not been able to function due to methylation cycle mutations it is as if it has accumulated cob-webs. It is important to get the cycle working gain, and the fastest route to do this is by supporting the "short cut" through the BHMT enzyme.

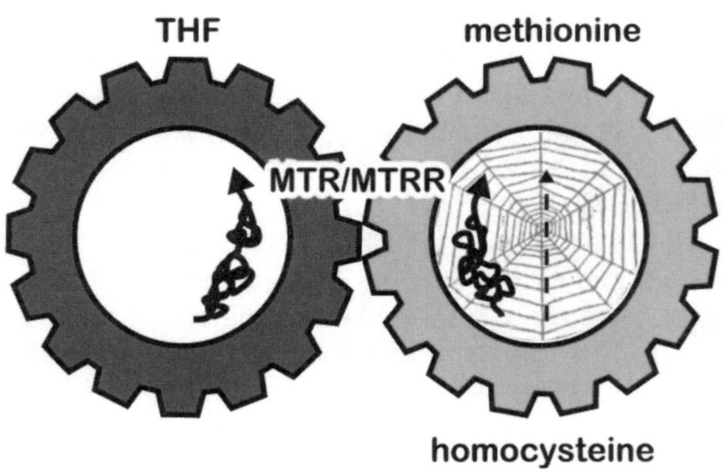

It is faster to support this backdoor reaction, or shortcut to get the cycle working again.

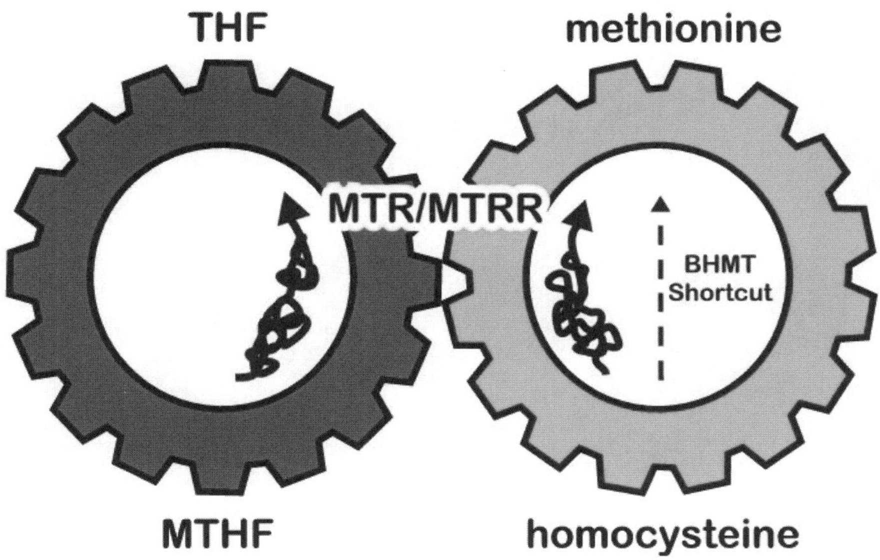

Over time, as you are able to support MTR, MTRR and MTHFR C677T mutations so that the long way around the cycle can function properly then the body will not need to rely as heavily on the shortcut through the BHMT enzyme. Once the methionine levels appear to be more in balance on a urine AA test, the methylmalonic acid levels are in normal range, and the FIGLU is in normal range it is time to consider looking at the use of DMG. The use of DMG is helpful in slowing the reaction through the BHMT enzyme and favoring the long way around the methylation cycle. Obviously it is essential to have supported any MTR, MTRR and MTHFR C677T mutations and run tests to look at pathway function before looking to make this shift.

There are some advantages to supporting the pathway so that you are able to go around the cycle, i.e. the “long way”, as well as having the ability to take the “short cut”. As a result I do think it is important to supplement with low doses of a range of supplements that support all of the weak points of the methylation cycle.

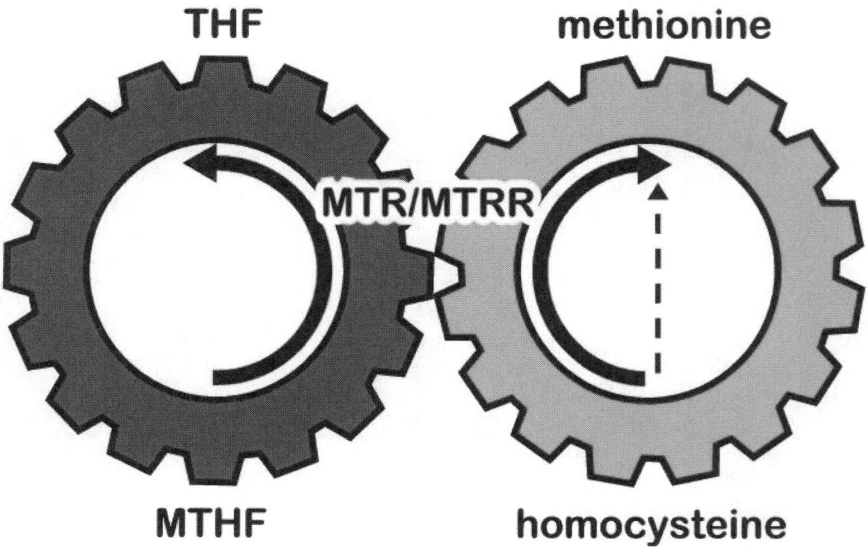

This would make sense as the building blocks for RNA and DNA are part of the reason you want to go the “long way” around the cycle. Using the BHMT enzyme to go from homocysteine to methionine will not help to generate RNA and DNA building blocks. This makes it difficult to repair new tissues or to expand T cell clones in response to infection. By adding RNA and nucleotides we take some of the pressure off the "long way" around the cycle so that we are not asking for as much activity via MTR and MTRR to generate the RNA and DNA building blocks. In a similar way by adding low dose folinic (1/4 Intrinsic B12 is the source for this) and low dose 5 methyl THF (1/4 Folapro) we help to supply additional intermediates that would normally be generated by the "long route" around the cycles. The nature of the MTHFR A1298C mutation suggests that supporting with Folapro will also help this enzyme to support adequate levels of BH4.

For individuals with CBS up regulations it is important that the CBS/ammonia situation be the primary starting point. To refresh your memory, the CBS enzyme basically acts as a gate between homocysteine and the rest of the transsulfuration pathway. While we normally think of mutations in terms of shutting off or decreasing enzyme function, these particular mutations increase the activity of the enzyme. Going back to the analogy with the gate, it is as if the gate is constantly open. This will allow support that we use for the rest of the methylation pathway to drain through the CBS enzyme into the transsulfuration pathway, including any B12 we add to address MTR and MTRR mutations or Folapro and Intrinsic to address MTHFR mutations. Unfortunately this "open gate" is not a neutral situation. While there are some positive end products that are generated via the transsulfuration pathway such as glutathione and taurine, there are also negative byproducts such as excess ammonia and sulfites. In order to detoxify this ammonia it requires the urea cycle, and uses BH4 that is needed for other functions in the body. In order to detoxify the sulfites it requires molybdenum. This leaves less molybdenum to help to address the zinc/copper ratio. In addition, manganese is also involved in ammonia detoxification as well as dopamine synthesis; an increased level of ammonia therefore reflects upon dopamine levels. On a related note, sulfur that is generated by all of the excess CBS activity has the ability to help to trigger this stress response. Chronic stress (the cortisol response) then up regulates the pathway via the BHMT enzyme. Until you get excess sulfur under control for the CBS mutations it may be necessary to add even more support for this alternate pathway (via the BHMT enzyme) early on, to prevent this aspect of the pathway from becoming depleted due to stress.

If you choose to utilize the Metals RNA Formulas you should work in conjunction with your health care provider. Start with 1/3 dropper Metals I RNA only 1X/day. You will continue at this low dosage for 2-3 weeks. "Overmethylated children" (COMT V158M + +, COMT H62H + +) represent the exception to the above-suggested dosages. Methylation is necessary to <u>prevent</u> the expression of viral genes that have been inserted into the body's DNA. Children who are overmethylated may therefore have lower viral loads than children who are "undermethylators" (COMT V158M - -). It is better to err on the side of "less is better" with respect to methylation with these children. Use 1/8 to 1/4 of the 5 methyl folate, intrinsic B12 and nucleotides for overmethylators, and use between 1/6 to 1/3 dropper of the RNA Metal formulas for these children.

Watch for signs of detoxification. These may include a rash, mild fever, mood changes, crankiness, and loose bowels. Occasionally children will vomit during this phase for no apparent reason, and then quickly resume their previous activity or even sit down for something to eat. This is all a part of the detoxification process. Several of the other RNA formulas may help to alleviate some of the discomfort associated with detoxification. It is fine to increase the dosage of the Health Foundation RNA Formula, the Stress RNA Formula, the Behavior RNA Formula, and the Nerve Calm RNA Formula or to use the Comfort Support. You may also want to try one or more of the Mood RNA formulas if your child is particularly moody during detoxification. If you experience more severe symptoms of detoxification, discontinue Step Two immediately. If you have questions during this phase of the program (or any other phases) please take advantage of the www.autismanswer.com website for online discussions and questions. In addition, it is recommended that you work with a qualified practitioner while following this protocol.

As you begin to experience detoxification, you will notice the urine getting darker. This can be monitored by weekly urine toxic metal tests. It is fine to take random spot urines some time in the mid afternoon. It is best to pick a day and time of the week to monitor and stick with that day and time weekly (i.e., Tuesday at 5:00 pm). You will notice that the creatinine numbers on the urine test will increase, as the urine gets darker. It is postulated that this represents viral detoxification in the urine. Eventually the urine will get lighter, almost clear. This is often when the metals begin to be excreted. You will be able to visualize this by continuing to take weekly urine samples. Over this time period you can begin to gradually increase the frequency of the Metal I RNA Formula. After 2-3 weeks of 1/3 dropper once a day, you can gradually increase to 1/3 dropper 2X/day for several days, then to 3X/day, up to 7-8X/day. As you increase the dosage of the Metal I RNA Formula you will notice increases in the creatinine (or color of the urine) followed by increases in the metal excretion. After you have reached a dosage of Metal I RNA Formula of 7-8 X/day for several weeks, and you are no longer seeing any excretion of metals, drop back to a maintenance dose of 1/3 dropper 1X/day. Occasionally, a child will appear to be almost "stuck" at this phase of detoxification. The urine remains dark, the creatinine continues to be high, and a very low but steady excretion of metals are seen on the urine tests. This is okay; every child is unique and may respond somewhat differently to the program. Just hang in there, don't feel rushed, and continue with the program until you finally see the urine clear and the metals begin to flow. While the average time for using Metal I at 7-8X/day is only a few weeks, we have seen children who required several months at this point. Realize that this program is not an "all or none" phenomena. You will see gradual changes as you progress through the program.

Once you have finished with Metals I, it is a good idea to give the body a rest for 2-4 weeks before going on to Metal II RNA Formula. It may be tempting to rush through the program once you begin to see metals and virus flowing. However, it is much easier on the system to give it time to rest between detoxification. In addition, it is often normal to see regressions in behavior and speech during detoxification. This can be scary for the parents. Giving a break between phases allows the behavior and the language to "bounce back", which is reassuring for everyone involved. With all of these caveats in mind, when you are ready, you can progress to Metal II RNA Formula.

This next phase of detoxification proceeds in basically the same fashion as the first phase. Continue with a maintenance dose of Metal I RNA Formula at 1/3 dropper 1X/day. You can then add the Metal II RNA Formula, starting with 1/3 dropper only 1X/day. You will continue at this low dosage for 2-3 weeks. After 2-3 weeks of 1/3 dropper once a day, you can gradually increase to 1/3 dropper 2X/day for several days, then to 3X/day, up to 7-8X/day. As you increase the dosage of the Metal II RNA Formula you will again notice increases in the creatinine (or color of the urine) followed by increases in the metal excretion. After you have reached a dosage of Metal II RNA Formula of 7-8X/day and you are no longer seeing any excretion of metals, drop back to a maintenance dose of 1/3 dropper 1X/day. At this point you will be using a maintenance dose of both Metal I RNA Formula and Metal II RNA Formula. Urines can be monitored during this second phase of detoxification as they were during the first phase. Again, at this point it is a good idea to give the body a rest for 2-4 weeks before going on to Metal III RNA Formula.

The third phase of detoxification proceeds basically the same as the first two phases. Continue with a maintenance dose of Metal I RNA Formula and Metal II RNA Formula at 1/3 dropper 1X/day for each. You can then add the Metal III RNA Formula, starting with 1/3 dropper only 1X/day. You will continue at this low dosage for 2-3 weeks. After 2-3 weeks of 1/3 dropper once a day, you can gradually increase to 1/3 dropper 2X/day for several days, then to 3X/day, up to 7-8X/day. As you increase the dosage of the Metal III RNA Formula you will again notice increases in the creatinine (or color of the urine) followed by increases in the metal excretion. After you have reached a dosage of Metal III RNA Formula of 7-8X/day for several weeks and you are no longer seeing any excretion of metals, drop back to a maintenance dose of 1/3 dropper 1X/day. At this point you will be using a maintenance dose of Metal I RNA Formula, Metal II RNA Formula and Metal III RNA Formula. Urines can be monitored during this third phase of detoxification as they were during the first two phases. Again, at this point it is a good idea to give the body a rest for 2-4 weeks before going on to Metal IV RNA Formula.

Weekly urine tests can get expensive, although the feedback is always gratifying for the parents. One trick is to watch for the color of the urine to get dark, and then get clear again. Simply send in the clear samples to try to get a measure of the metal excretion. This will not monitor creatinine and potential viral excretion, and you may miss some metals, but it will be easier on the budget. A number of parents have taken advantage of the creatinine test strips. While these strips are not quantitative, they will give you a sense of the trend of the creatinine numbers. By using the creatinine test strips in conjunction with biweekly (or every third week) spot urine tests you can follow the urine metal excretion as suggested in a more cost effective manner. It should be noted that aluminum excretion appears to be independent of the creatinine number, unlike mercury or lead. For this reason it is important not to rely solely on the creatinine test strips to determine when to send in a spot urine sample for toxic metals. Sending in spot urine samples should be done on a regular basis, even if the creatinine numbers have not dropped to indicate a clearing of the urine color. In addition, the use of spot urine essential minerals along with the toxic metal excretion is very important. The essential minerals can be excreted along with toxic metals. Depletions of essential minerals can be a cause for concern. For this reason alone, you should take occasional spot urine tests regardless of the creatinine number and ALSO include a check of essential minerals.

After a sufficient rest following Metals I, II, III it is time to progress to Metals IV. At this point you will be using a maintenance dose of Metal I RNA Formula, Metal II RNA Formula and Metal III RNA Formula. This next phase of detoxification using Metals IV proceeds in basically the same fashion as the previous phases. Continue with the maintenance doses of Metals I, II, and III RNA Formulas at 1/3 dropper 1X/day. You can then add the Metal IV RNA Formula, starting with 1/3 dropper only 1X/day. You will continue at this low dosage for 2-3 weeks. After 2-3 weeks of 1/3 dropper once a day, you can gradually increase to 1/3 dropper 2X/day for several days, then to 3X/day, up to 7-8X/day. After you have reached a dosage of Metal IV RNA Formula of 7-8X/day and you are no longer seeing any excretion of metals, drop back to a maintenance dose of 1/3 dropper 1X/day. During this final phase of detoxification metals are often excreted in the stool as well as the urine. Stools should be monitored during this final phase of detoxification. Urine tests can be continued, however, stool toxic analysis has proven useful at this stage of detoxification. In addition the skin rash can be more visible at this time.

Frequent baths are a good idea at this stage of detoxification. The bath should contain EDTA (Beyond Clean) and may also contain malic acid, and oatmeal or Aveeno to relieve itching. The Health Foundation RNA as well as the HyperImmune Formula may also be useful used topically at this point. In addition, the Topical Skin Formula is also helpful, as well as any topical creams including glutathione (this is a sulfur donor, look at genetics), horse chestnut, aloe, MSM (this is both a methyl and sulfur donor, so look at genetics). Saunas may be helpful to accelerate detoxification through the skin. The use of saunas to accelerate toxin release has been thoroughly described by Dr. Stephen Edelson. Metals IV can be applied topically as a cosmetic prior to taking a sauna to enhance absorption.

There have been mixed reports concerning the use of Vitamin A to aid in eradicating chronic viral infection. Some parents choose to add 100,000 IU of Vitamin A every other day for a period of 2 weeks as a concentrated approach to aiding in recovery from virus. In addition, some protocols use prescription antivirals, such as Valtrex in conjunction with the Metal IV portion of the detoxification program. It is also worth considering the use of Valtrex in conjunction with the use of Depakane (valproic acid). Valproic acid can be used to treat seizures. There is literature to suggest that valproic acid may exacerbate measles viral infection. Subsequent research has found the combination of Valtrex in conjunction with depakane to be beneficial.

It is normal to see rashes, a mild fever, and regression in behavior during detoxification. Occasionally, parents have reported that their child may vomit, for no particular reason, during this phase, and then calmly resume their activity or even sit down for something to eat with no ill effects. This may be part of the detoxification process. At any point during the detoxification program that you are concerned about behaviors, the extent of detoxification, rashes, fever, or other physical symptoms simply stop the program and those symptoms will subside in several days. You can go back to the program at any point and restart. Simply remember to begin again at a dose of 1X/day, and gradually work your way up.

Some parents have looked at a combination detoxification support as a final "clean up" of Step 2. This combination includes the use of Metals I, Metals IV, Microbial Support RNAs along with Valtrex. In a similar fashion as described above, the amount of the Metals I, IV and Microbial Support are gradually increased over time. This combination approach is only used after each of the Metals RNAs has first been used individually as described above. Again, detoxification should always be conducted in conjunction with your health care provider.

Some parents like to accelerate the detoxification program. This can be accomplished by increasing the dosage of some of the other supplements. For instance, during Step One (Program for Neurological Inflammation) we used a maintenance dose of EDTA once a day, and additional garlic once a day. During Step Two, the detoxification part of the program the dosages of EDTA and garlic can be gradually increased to aid in accelerating the process. Also don't forget to continue with nightly baths using the EDTA Beyond Clean formula. This will aid in detoxification through the skin. A number of parents have also chosen to combine saunas with the detoxification portion of the protocol, again to help accelerate the detoxification.

It is important to keep the concept of the total body burden of metals and chemicals in mind during detoxification. There has understandably been a tremendous emphasis on mercury with respect to elimination. However, toxic levels of lead, aluminum and other metals can be just as dangerous. Cadmium has the ability to enhance the toxic level of lead, making lower levels of lead more toxic in the presence of cadmium. We have seen children excrete exceedingly high levels of uranium and tin (see sample detox data). One can only speculate as to the cumulative effects of these metal levels in conjunction with only minor levels of mercury.

We therefore need to consider the synergistic total burden on the body. We have noted some interesting kinetics in terms of metal excretion in urine. We have observed that nickel is often excreted prior to mercury, and that cadmium excretion often precedes that of lead. The kinetics of metal excretion will continue to be clarified in the future, and we will adjust this protocol to reflect future findings. We continue to evolve our detoxification protocol, and an additional detoxification step, Metals V, is available

As already mentioned, it is important to keep essential minerals in balance while you are excreting toxic metals. Dr. Yasko has observed that lithium and iodine levels tend to drop along with the excretion of mercury. In similar manner calcium, strontium and boron tend to decrease with the excretion of lead. Again, the excretion of nickel and cadmium signal the future excretion of mercury and lead respectively. Therefore the excretion of nickel can be used as a sign to anticipate excretion of mercury and to keep an eye on lithium and iodine levels. In an analogous fashion, the excretion of cadmium predicts the future excretion of lead and suggests that you monitor the levels of calcium, boron and strontium more closely.

Step 2: Suggested Protocol to Support Detoxification

Vitamins/ Minerals/ Antioxidants to Lay the Nutritional Groundwork:

Cell Food/BioNativus Multimins
Selenium
Molybdenum
Complete Vitamin & Ultra Antioxidant
Vitamin D
Nerve Calm RNA Formula
Health Foundation RNA Formula
Stress RNA Formula
HyperImmune RNA Formula (limited us for COMT+)
Behavior RNA Formula
Bowel RNA Formula
Stomach pH RNA Formula

Supplements to Support Viral Detoxification:

Metal I RNA Formula (progress to Metals II, III, IV, V)
FolaPro (5 methyl folate)
Intrinsic B12/Folate
Folinic
Nucleotides
Elderberry (increase to 4 to 6 per day)
Garlic (LIMITED FOR CBS+) start with 1X/day, may increase up to 6X/day
Policosanol
Glutathione (LIMITED FOR CBS+) 1X/day, then increase to 4 or more per day)
L-Lysine
Melissa
Moducare (start 1X in AM and 1X in PM, increase to 4X/day)
EDTA (start with 1X/day, may increase to 4-6X/day)
Beyond Clean EDTA bath- nightly
Colostrum (start with 1X/day, then increase to 2-3X/day)
Alpha Lipoic Acid (LIMITED for CBS+ and MTHFR A1298C)
Vitamin C

Synthetic B1 (Benfotiamine)
Transfer Factor
Cats Claw
Aloe Vera
Quercetin (LIMITED for COMT V158M+)
Proline
IMF 4 (with Metals I, II, III)
IMF 1, 2, 6 (with Metals IV)

Supplements to Support the Immune System/ Increase White Cells:

Transfer Factor
IP6
MGN3
Mycoceutics (mushrooms/beta glucan)
Pau d Arco
Ayur-Guggulipid
Myrrh Gum
Fenugreek
SerenAid (start with 1/4 per day, increase to 1/2 or 1X/day)
Lactoferrin (every other day)
L-Theanine
IMFs

Supplements to Help Support the Liver/ Pancreas/ Thymus/ Spleen:

Ora -Triplex
Immuno-Forte
Ora-Liv
Ora-Pancreas
Cod Liver Oil
SAMe
B Complex
Ora-Kidney

Support Oxygenation/ Alkalinity to Limit Viral Growth:

- Oxydrene
- O2 Plus
- Penta water
- ATP
- Cell Food
- Ionic Breeze (Sharper Image)
- pH Kit and balancing for alkaline pH

Optional:

- Vitamin A (100,000 IU every other day for 2 weeks)
- Valtrex
- Bone Support RNA

Note: *If supplements are listed in more than one category the intention is to take the supplement only once a day. They are listed in each category to give a sense of the multiple uses of the individual supplements.*

Use of OAT/MAT & Urine AA Tests to Monitor Status of Bypassing Methylation Cycle Mutations

Indications of **CBS Up Regulations**:

Urine AA Test

Elevated taurine
Elevated ammonia
Decreased citrulline
Decreased methionine
Elevated phenylalanine

OAT/MAT

Elevated hippuric
Decreased fumarate
Elevated phenyl lactate, phenyl acetate, phenylethylamine
Decreased oxaloacetate or decreased oxalates
(Secondary to decreased oxalate you can find elevated hydroxymethylglutarate and elevated hydroxybutyrate. Elevated ammonia requires more urea cycle function, depleting oxaloacetate from the Krebs cycle. Imbalances in oxaloacetate can lead to an increase in the level of hydroxybutyrate.)
Blood work
Low CO_2
Low creatinine

You may not see changes in these values with CBS up regulations until you begin to supplement the methylation cycle to bypass other mutations in the pathway.

Indications of **Decreased Methylation Cycle Function**:

Urine AA Test

Low methionine on a urine AA test
Elevated methylhistidine

OAT/MAT

Increased FIGLU
Increased methylmalonic acid
Low succinic
High uracil relative to thymidine
Elevations in beta amino isobutyrate and anserine
(Can be produced by excess uracil that is not processed to thymidine due to lack of methyl groups.)

Elevated methyl histidine, FIGLU and uracil reflect the fact that the methylation cycle is not supported fully. High methylmalonic and low succinic more specifically look at B12 levels.

If the methylation cycle is not supplemented properly it may be difficult to get an accurate measure of B12 levels. You will not begin to use B12 at appreciable levels until the other mutations in the pathway have been bypassed with nutritional support. For this reason, methylmalonic and succinic levels may appear to be in range until you have added the rest of the methylation cycle support. If methylmalonic and succinic are in range, yet FIGLU is high, methionine is low and taurine is elevated, I suggest that you supplement to bypass mutations and then rerun to test for methylmalonic and succinic levels.

If you have been supporting to bypass mutations and the MMA and succinic are in range and FIGLU is still high then you may need increased levels of plain folate. The use of the HHC general should support this need. As an alternative, or in addition, look at increasing your use of Intrinsic B12 relative to Folapro (i.e., every other day use 1/4 Intrinsic B12 twice daily rather than 1/4 Folapro and 1/4 Intrinsic B12 every day).

High levels of methionine sulfoxide may indicate a need for additional ATP. High levels of methionine as well as methionine sulfoxide with sufficient ATP support may suggest decreased MAT enzyme activity and the need to support directly with SAMe, regardless of the COMT and VDR status to bypass MAT (methionine adenosyl transferase) mutations.

Indications that you **have addressed the CBS up regulations are a drop in ammonia, decreased taurine and an increase in creatinine, signaling the start of detoxification**:

- Urine AA test
  - Decreased ammonia
  - Increased creatinine
  - Decreased taurine
  - Increased sarcosine
  - Secondary to increased oxalates:
    - Increased beta alanine
    - Increased beta amino isobutyrate
    - Increased carnosine
    - Increased anserine

- OAT/MAT test
  - Elevated oxaloacetate
  - Elevated oxalates

When you begin to address CBS up regulations with the ammonia program the ammonia levels will drop allowing creatinine to increase. Elevated creatinine and elevated aspartate due to decreased ammonia/urea cycle activity can lead to increased beta alanine and carnosine as this is another way to get rid of the excess. With decreased ammonia, arginine from the urea cycle is available to produce creatinine. This can cause increased levels of aspartate. Aspartate can then feed into the Krebs cycle to increase the level of oxaloacetate. Aspartate can also result in elevated beta alanine. Beta alanine leads to increased levels of carnosine and anserine. (High level support for the "short cut" can also result in elevations of beta alanine, carnosine and anserine.)

Indications that **Support for "Short Cut" Through BHMT is High**:

- Elevated glycine
- Elevated sarcosine
- Elevated phosphatidyl serine

Initially it can be visualized as if the methylation cycle is inactive and full of cobwebs. If there are mutations in MTR and/or MTRR, then support for the BHMT pathway is necessary to get the methylation cycle moving; increases in sarcosine and glycine may occur. As creatinine decreases sarcosine can be seen to increase.

Rhodiola inhibits creatinine kinase. The use of rhodiola may lead to increased levels of sarcosine and glycine on amino acid tests.

Indications of **Decreased BH4**:

High hippuric
Increased 8 hydroxy 2 deoxy guanosine
(lack of SAMe or high ammonia can also cause increased 8 hydroxy 2 deoxy guanosine)
Elevated phenylalanine, phenyl lactate, phenyl acetate, phenylethylamine
Increased ammonia

Increased **VMA and HVA**:

The breakdown of dopamine results in HVA. The breakdown of norepinephrine results in VMA. When there is excessive support for the BHMT enzyme we can often see higher VMA relative to HVA on a MAT/OAT test. This may suggest that it is time to add in DMG and/or SAMe to help to support a shift to the longer route around the methylation cycle. Obviously you need to have addressed the CBS issues and have adequate support for any MTR/MTRR/MTHFR mutations before you can consider this shift. Recall that once the methionine levels appear to be more in balance on a urine AA test, and the methylmalonic acid, succinic, taurine and FIGLU are in normal range it is time to consider looking at the use of DMG. The use of DMG is helpful in slowing the reaction through the BHMT enzyme and favoring the long way around the methylation cycle. Obviously it is essential to have supported any MTR, MTRR and MTHFR C677T mutations and run tests to look at pathway function before looking to make this shift.

On the other hand high levels of HVA indicate increased breakdown of dopamine. You should consider using low dose Mood

D, quercetin and/or Mood Focus to help to keep dopamine levels in the normal healthy range.

Indications of **Decreased Urea Cycle/OTC Activity**:

High fumarate
Midrange/high ornithine
Midrange/high arginine
Low aspartate
Low malic acid
Low citrulline

Low urea cycle/OTC activity can result from decreased methylation cycle function. If FIGLU is high, methylmalonic is high, succinic is low and methionine is low it also indicates that methylation cycle support is needed in addition to OTC support.

OAT tests and MAT tests are extremely valuable tools in helping to monitor how well nutritional support is working to bypass mutations in nutritional pathways. However, I feel that a CDSA with sensitivity testing is the ultimate tool for determining if bacteria or yeast is a problem in the gut. A direct toxin stool test can be used to screen for *Clostridia*.

Step 3: Program for Nerve Growth & Myelination

This is the phase that everyone has been waiting for. Unfortunately, there is still a bit more waiting even during this phase. It can take up to nine months to remyelinate the nerves that have been demyelinated from virus, metals, and other assaults to the system. Once the nerves are remyelinated they are finally in a position to begin the "pruning" process. This also takes time. The exception to this is children who are "over methylators". This process will occur much more rapidly for children who tend to be over methylated.

The methylation pathway is also tied into the pathways for neurotransmitters. As a result, you may see changes in mood and behaviors as you go through this phase. Initially many parents will comment that the child is "no longer autistic" but "acts more like a child with ADD". This makes sense as dopamine has been implicated in ADD as well as in the methylation process. The Mood RNA Formulas can be very helpful at this stage. There are three Mood Formulas. Depending on the particular child one or more of these Formulas may be helpful. A good starting point is to use 1/3 dropper of one of the formulas for several days, then make a decision on that formula before switching to a different formula or adding a second formula for a combined effect. Also, some parents have seen great things with small amounts of supplements containing natural dopamine. Also, as described in a prior section of this book, imbalances in the level of norepinephrine relative to dopamine can cause some of the hyperactivity and attention issues that have been described. Looking to balance support for the "long way" around the pathway relative to the "short cut" through the methylation cycle is very helpful in getting the behaviors back in balance. In addition, looking at the ratio of VMA to HVA also described above while help to guide you in this process.

At this point, depending on the calcium levels seen on a urine essential element test, you may want to look at adding calcium back. It will aid in neurotransmission; however, too much calcium can still be a problem. One approach is to use a calcium/ magnesium/vitamin D/vitamin K supplement, and substitute it for the individual magnesium, vitamin D and vitamin K supplements. Again, this will vary depending on the child and on the level of calcium in the system.

It is possible to accelerate the myelination process somewhat by using higher dosages of some of the supplements that support myelination. Some parents have used up to four SAMe per day with two B complex. In addition, they have used two curcumin and doubled up on some of the other methylating agents. While this may speed up the process, watch carefully for potential side effects such as mood swings or vision issues. If this occurs, back off on the dosages. Do NOT increase the levels of 5 methyl folate, intrinsic, folinic, or the nucleotides. Due to the MTHFr mutation in virtually all of the children, this could create problems. You are better off to just keep the door open on this MTHFr pathway, rather than flooding it with supplementation. B12 deserves special mention in terms of dosage. So far, according to published work by Dr. Neubrander, no toxic doses of B12 have been found. The more the better seems to be what parents are finding. In some cases going to highly elevated doses of B12 (50 milligrams and above) has helped to stimulate speech in children that were apraxic. However, it is always possible that your child will be the one child who will react adversely to high doses of B12. Again, progress slowly, use caution, and consult with your health care practitioner when utilizing this or any other program. Children who are "overmethylators" are the exception. These children cannot tolerate high doses of any methylating agents, so caution and low doses should be used when supplementing these children with methylating agents. A knowledge of the nutrigenomic profile is very useful with respect to B12 support. It can help you to determine if hydroxy or methyl B12 would better suit your child. Nutrigenomics will also help you to gauge to amount of B12 that may be needed to achieve balance in the system.

The major focus of this final phase of the program involves supplements to support remyelination of the nerves and supplements to foster left/right communication in the brain. Many of the supplements used in the previous phases can be discontinued at this time. The approach to discontinuing supplements should be very similar to the approach used to add supplements. Eliminate several supplements at a time, and then wait to be sure that you are not seeing regressions as a result of discontinuing supplements. Go back to the categories listed in Step One, and try to keep in some support from each category. Even though we may have detoxified virus and metals, there are still many of the underlying factors discussed in the earlier portions of this book. The idea is to keep enough supplementation in the program to prevent this entire process from happening all over again. No one wants that to happen! So, while you may be tempted to only use the supplements listed in Step Three for Nerve Growth and Myelination, remember where you have been. It is a lot easier to give a little bit of a large number of supplements daily, then to run the risk of glutamate, viral and metal toxin buildup occurring again.

You may want to consider incorporating the use of magnetic therapy at this time. The basic premise for the use of magnetic devices is that the human body responds to the influence of the Earth's magnetic field. However, the strength of this field has decreased over time. In certain individuals this lack of magnetism can cause deficiencies, which can be improved by the use of external applications of magnetic fields.

Applications of magnetic fields have been successful in diverse situations, affecting specific chemical reactions (Grenoble High Magnetic Field Laboratory and the Max Planck Society) to the reduction of pain. In laboratory animals, magnets can act like a switch to open or constrict blood vessels, potentially increasing blood flow to damaged tissues. Pulsed electromagnetic fields have been shown to reduce bone resorption, and increase vascularization and bone formation. The use of magnetized water (Nariwa) is reported to aid in the excretion of mercury.

While Dr. Yasko has not found the use of magnetic energy to enhance metal excretion, she has seen a significant discernable affect on more subtle cognitive function. This would agree with recent work by Dr. Dean Bonlie, which has found electromagnetic therapy to be safe and effective for a wide range of neurological problems and that it may help to regenerate and repair damaged nerves and enhance the body's natural stem cells. Magnetic energy may also increase the oxygen carrying capacity of the blood, improving the assimilation of nutrients and oxygenation of tissues. The use of Nariwa magnetized water, and Penta oxygenated water may also be useful adjuncts to any program to enhance nerve growth and demyelination.

This is also a point where it would make sense to begin to integrate therapies that enhance nerve growth and maturation. The March 2004 issue of the Journal of Neuroscience describes significant increases in the levels of BDNF (brain derived neurotrophic factor) depending on the environment; an enriched environment fostered higher levels of this factor. BDNF promotes neuronal growth and survival and regulates communication between neurons. Dr. Cheri Florence, a medical speech/language pathologist, has described tremendous personal success with her own son. She has made use of strategies, which may help to create an enriched environment, by taking advantage of enhanced visual thinking to help promote language.

Dr. David Steenblock, Dr. Barbara Brewitt and Dr. Luis Aguilar have pioneered the direct use of some of these brain growth factors for stroke as well as autism, among others. Insulin like growth factor (IGF) has been found to stimulate enzymes in the methylation pathway in addition to its effects on neural development. Fibroblast growth factor (FgF) has also been found to have activities beyond its effects on nerve growth; FgF has been reported to increase dopamine levels, as well as to decrease seizure activity.

Dr. Edward Traub has developed CI (constraint induced) Movement therapy, which has proven to expedite recovery times after stroke. The basis of the therapy is helping the brain to overcome "learned non-use". Some of these therapies may be applicable to autism in the future to help to accelerate recovery after the biochemical imbalances have been addressed.

Music therapy has been reported to be successful in helping to enhance speech in children. A number of scientific journals have found that music affects regions of the brain involved in cognitive, affective and mnemonic processing. The entire July 2003 issue of Nature Neuroscience was devoted to music and neuroscience, as was the March 2004 issue of the New York Academy of Sciences magazine. Recent research from the University of London suggests that many autistic children have outstanding abilities in tone memory and discrimination. Music therapy may be an avenue worth exploring to help to enhance language skills during this point of the program.

Step 3: Suggested Protocol to Support Nerve Growth & Myelination

General Vitamin/ Organ Support:

- Complete Vitamin & Ultra Antioxidant
- Liquid Trace Minerals
- Ora-Liv
- Ora-Pancreas
- Ora-Triplex
- Immuno-Forte
- Cod Liver Oil
- Zinc
- Potassium chloride (depending on levels)
- Nerve Calm RNA Formula
- Health Foundation RNA Formula
- Stress RNA Formula
- Nerve Coat RNA Formula
- Behavior RNA Formula
- Bowel RNA Formula
- Stomach pH RNA Formula

Support Nutrient Transport to Brain (taken with supplements):

- Vitamin C (PLAIN Beyond C with no MSM)

Support Methylation (increases myelin):

- Curcumin
- SAMe
- B12 (balance of methyl/cyano/hydroxy cobalamine)
- Intrinsic B12/Folate
- FolaPro (5 Methyl Folate)
- Folinic
- Nucleotides
- DMG
- B Complex
- Selenium (up to 100-200mcg/day incl. Complete Vitamins)
- Amino Care amino acids
- MSM (depending on CBS status)

Support Myelination/ Cell Membranes Fluidity:

- DHA (100-600mg/day)
- Phosphatidyl serine
- Nerve Coat RNA (1/2 dropper 2X/day or as needed)
- EFA
- Policosanol
- Chondroitin sulfate (high MW) (LIMITED for CBS+)
- Glucosamine sulfate (LIMITED for CBS+)
- Sphingolin

Help Limit ROS (which triggers macrophage digestion of myelin):

- CoQ10
- Alpha Lipoic Acid (LIMITED for CBS+)
- Idebenone
- Vitamin E +mixed tocopherols
- Quercetin (LIMITED for COMT+)

Limit Macrophage Digestion of Myelin (MAY be an issue for phenol sensitive):

- Flavinoids:
    - Lutein/Bilberry
    - Quercetin

Pycnogenol
Grape Seed extract
Elderberry
Cranberry
Green Tea or L-Theanine

Support New Nerve Growth/ Support Nerves:

Ashwaganda
SAMe
B12
Milk thistle
B complex
Colostrum
IGF
FGF
HGH
Taurine
Ora-Placenta
Ginkgo Biloba
Carnosine
Rosemary
DHEA (monitor with hormone test)
Synthetic B1 (benfotiamine)
Shark liver oil (nervonic acid)
Vitamin K (or vit d/k/ca/mg depending on calcium levels)
Vitamin D (or vit d/k/ca/mg depending on calcium levels)
Magnesium (or vit d/k/ca/mg depending on calcium levels)
Calcium- *DEPENDING ON CALCIUM LEVELS*
L-Tyrosine
Glutathione (LIMITED for CBS+)
Choline, or lecithin, or huperzine (depending on the child)

Supplements to Support Progesterone for Nerve Growth:

GABA
Sublingual GABA Calm/ Glycine
Zen

Support Oxygenation/ Energy for New Nerve Growth:

- Oxydrene
- ATP
- Carnitine/acetyl-carnitine
- Vinpocetine
- NADH
- Cell Food
- Magnetico Magnetic Mattress (north only, 20 gauss)
- Body Fields OMT Magnopro
- Ionic Breeze (Sharper Image)
- Penta water
- Hyperbaric oxygen
- Nariwa water
- O2 Plus

Supplements to Support Moods:

- Mood-S Formula
- Mood-D Formula
- Mood & Focus Formula
- Dopa 400

Support Language:

- DMG
- Fenugreek (start with 1X/day increase to 3X/day)
- Gotu Kola
- Bacopa
- Piracetam
- B12-cyano/methyl/hydroxy cobalamin
- Black Cohosh
- Dong Quai
- Indole 3 Carbinol (discontinue if a fish odor from the body)
- Spinal Nerve Support RNA Formula

Supplements to Support Left/ Right Communication:

- Gotu Kola
- Bacopa

Nootropics:
- Piracetam
- Aniracetam

Fenugreek
Creatine

Supplements to Keep Virus in Check (IF still an issue):
- Transfer Factor
- Moducare (may increase gamma interferon)
- Glutathione
- Metals I, II, III, IV RNA Formulas

Note: *If supplements are listed in more than one category the intention is to take the supplement only once a day. They are listed in each category to give a sense of the multiple uses of the individual supplements.*

Conclusion: *A Ship in the Storm*

"At 13 months we were traveling with our son in Europe and people would stop us and say, "Look how he looks at you, the love in his eyes." By 18 months he no longer knew who we were, was unable to look at us and had lost all his language (he was speaking English and Spanish words). The pediatrician told us "Yes, 18 months is when Autism/PDD begins".

As parents, pregnant with twin boys at the time, we began frantically researching and traveling all over the US, meeting with DAN doctors, going to conferences etc. The physicians we met with, all had a piece of the puzzle and our son began to show improvements but we were far from recovery.

At 3 years old we still had no language so we taught Matthew to sign for things he needed. He still had many sensory issues; repetitive behavior couldn't sleep at night and would have terrible tantrums.

At the DAN conference in Boston 2002 I met some mothers from New York and they invited me to a meeting they have once a month at Jacobi Hospital. My husband and I went and we sat next to a mom who was talking about the success she was having with this "Dr. Amy" in Maine. She had been through the circuit of DAN doctors that we were now going to, and told us "Amy has figured it out".

I called Amy the next day and got an appointment within the next few weeks. We feel blessed because now we would have to wait quite some time, and that is why this book is so important.

Amy spent two hours on the phone with us on our initial consult. My husband is an MD and he was blown away by Amy's intelligence and dedication. He was also a bit skeptical about the supplements she was recommending because he was not trained that way. We began her protocol anyway.

Matthew continued to recover everyday with Amy's protocol; we also used Dr. Gordon's EDTA to slowly chelate him. In July of 2003, Amy sent us the detoxification phase of the protocol. One month later Matthew began excreting high levels of mercury and other metals. By the middle of September, Matthew walked in our kitchen and asked in a perfect sentence "could he have a glass of water". We almost fell on the floor.

Matthew just turned 5 in June 2004. He just graduated from Preschool, and he was the star of the show. He has incredible language and loves to play with other kids. He no longer has repetitive behavior and will be going to kindergarten in September. He loves to have sleepovers with his friends and with his cousins.

We are about 95% recovered from that deep dark world that Matthew was stuck in. We are now in the fine tuning phase. Our twin boys are now 2 years 7 months. We now have three healthy beautiful little boys.

We are so happy that Amy and Dr. Gordon have decided to publish a book on the protocols so other families can get started. It is a long but rewarding journey for everyone involved. Amy will continue to research and educate the parents to give them the knowledge to recover the children. Through this process she has rescued Matthew and saved my other two sons from going down that dreadful dark ally. We are truly grateful to her."

Marilyn M. and Dr. John M., Parents of Matthew, age 5

Now you have read through the protocols and can't wait to get started. That is excellent. Any parent or physician reading this should be excited and hopeful. This protocol has been a tremendous benefit to a number of children. It has worked for children of all ages, and no, this protocol does not require that your child be less than 5 years old. Individuals up to 30 years of age have seen benefits from this program. However, it is not a magic bullet. For most children there is no magic bullet. It is a matter of perseverance, and slowly working your way through the program to gradually reverse the layers of damage, and put all of the complex pieces back together and in working order. Yes, it can be done, and it has been done. There are always the "quick fix" kids; the ones that need only a few supplements or just the first phase of the detoxification program to be on their way to recovery. We all hear about those cases, and it seems like everyone except YOUR child falls into that category. Well, the reality is that most children do not fall into the quick fix category. But there is hope for every child. So, take a deep breath, get ready for the marathon, pace yourself, but above all else don't give up on your children.

One way to think about neurological inflammation is like a ship that is drifting out to sea, being carried further and further from shore by the tide. Out of nowhere, a rope is thrown to that ship. First, all that happens is the ship stops moving out to sea with the tide. It seems like nothing is happening and all is still lost. However, the very fact that the ship is no longer moving, that it is staying in place, means that the movement out to sea has been stopped, that the direction is reversed, and the progression of the disease has been halted. Then slowly the ship begins to move back toward the shore. It moves very slowly because it moves against the tide working to pull it back out to sea. Over time, the ship moves closer and closer to the land until finally, when you least expect it, there it is, safe on the shore. Hold on tight to your rope, don't lose hope; it truly is possible to recover your children.

With love and hope for the future,

Dr. Amy Yasko and Dr. Garry Gordon

Additional Suggested Resources
for Parents and Practitioners

Anglesey, Deborah Battling the MSG Myth. Front Porch Press www.msgmyth.com

Blaylock, Russell L. New Developments in the Prevention and Treatment of Neurodegenerative Diseases. *JANA* 5 (2002): 15-32.

Blaylock, Russell L. Excitotoxins: The Taste that Kills. Santa Fe, New Mexico: Health P, 1997.

Blaylock R. The Central Role of Excitotoxicity in Autism Spectrum Disorders. *JANA* 2003; 6(1): 10.

Blaylock R. Interaction of Cytokines, Excitotoxins, and Reactive Nitrogen and Oxygen Species in Autism Spectrum Disorders. *JANA* 2003; 6(4): 21.

Gordon G. The Omega-3 Miracle. Freedom Press, 2004

Yasko A. & Gordon G. Heal Your Body Naturally: The Power of RNA. Matrix Development Publishing, 2004.

Yasko A. Genetic Bypass. Matrix Development Publishing, 2005.

There are several basic videos that are available that help to lay the groundwork for the autism program. These include the ***Neurological Inflammation*** video and the ***Putting It All Together*** video.

Dr. Yasko suggests watching the ***Neurological Inflammation*** video first. The Neurological Inflammation tape is the most basic and most general. It explains the glutamate/GABA and excitotoxin issue in more detail than any of the subsequent tapes. There is a slight noise in the background of this tape. There was an autistic child putting pennies into a bank while Dr. Amy spoke for 3 hours. She was impressed with his attentiveness and was happy to have him there and was not about to ask him to stop putting pennies in the bank or ask him to leave to improve the audio on a tape. So please think of it as a happy noise rather than as an annoyance.

The next video in complexity is the ***Putting It All Together*** two VHS tape or DVD set that was recorded at a weekend workshop in January, 2004. This video includes a round table discussion with some very well informed parents of autistic children that is extremely useful. This video will help you to comprehend some of the topics that are covered in more scientific detail in the ***Boston DVDs***. Furthermore, these videos slowly lay the groundwork for the autism book, ***The Puzzle of Autism: Putting It All Together***.

The ***Boston Conference*** DVD set from August 2004 would be the next resource to study. If you had a chance to read the "The Motivation" section of the book, Dr. Yasko explained that we published this book about a year before we would have liked to in order to get the protocol in your hands as soon as possible. As a result the book does not contain all of the scientific detail she and Dr. Gordon would have otherwise included. There was not the time to put in the kind of detailed information they would have liked and still publish the book in a timely fashion. What we did to address this need was to host the two day conference in Boston in August just as the book was released. This conference covered the protocol in detail. It is highly suggested that you get the DVDs from this conference and watch them. The DVDs should help to answer a tremendous number of questions. By the time you have finished watching these videos you will have a much, much better grasp of the program.

Next, there is ***Dr. Amy's Supplement Guide*** video that was taped over Christmas break, 2004. In this 3 hour video Dr. Yasko goes over each supplement listed in the book and explains her personal rationale for the use of these supplements when designing a custom supplement plan for a child. This video is an excellent tool for putting together a supplement plan for Step 1 of the program. The more recent use of nutrigenomic testing in her practice and the custom Genetic Analysis Review (GAR) supplement programs that she writes up based on these results are basically the beginning of Step 2 of the program. Therefore it may be useful to review ***Dr. Amy's Supplement Guide*** if you have not already done so, to be certain that you have included any of the needed supplements for organ support as part of Step 1 before embarking on Step 2 with the suggestions in a GAR. This video also begins to touch upon the role that nutrigenomics play in putting together a supplement plan.

The role of nutrigenomics testing in developing individualized supplement plans was a topic that was covered comprehensively in the April 2005 conference in Phoenix, Arizona as ***Personalized Medicine***. This topic was also covered in both the May 2005 ACAM presentation, ***Implications of Genetic Testing for Alternative Healthcare***, as well as the November 2005 ACAM conference presentation, ***Nutrigenomics, Methylation, and RNA Based Nutrients.***

All of Dr. Yasko's programs rely heavily on the use of RNA supplements. It is useful to understand why RNA is so important for certain conditions, and the way in which it functions in the body because they are so central to the program. The RNA book, ***Heal Your Body Naturally: The Power of RNA***, explains the background for the use of RNA. It is written in laymen's terms so that anyone really can understand it. There is a short video available concerning the use of nutritional RNAs, ***RNA Regulation***; the use of RNA is also covered on the ***Boston Conference*** DVDs. This topic was also covered in detail during the April 2005 conference in the presentations ***Why Do We Need RNA?*** and ***Understanding the Use of RNA***. The complete DVD set from the April 2005 conference includes the talk on ***Personalized Medicine***, the two talks concerning the use of RNA, as well as a several hour talk on ***Microbes, Metals and Methylation***.

Finally, watch for the upcoming DVD set from the ***February 2006 Phoenix Conference***. This was a full two-day conference covering topics ranging from Nutrigenomics, Metals and Microbes to Glutamate and GABA.

Resources Divided by Topic

Glutamate and Gaba
Neurological Inflammation – VHS or DVD Set
Phoenix Conference, February 2006 – DVD Set
CASD Conference, November 2004 – DVD Set
Phoenix Conference, April 2005 – DVD Set
Phoenix Conference, February 2006 – DVD Set

Factors Contributing to Autism
Putting It All Together Parents Weekend - VHS or DVD Set
Boston Conference, August 2004 – DVD Set
The Puzzle of Autism - Book
Autism Educational Starter Packet (ESP) – DVD Set & Book
Dr. Amy's Supplement Guide - DVD Set
Phoenix Conference, February 2006 – DVD Set

RNA
Boston Conference, August 2004 – DVD Set
Phoenix Conference, April 2005 – DVD Set
Heal Your Body Naturally – Book
RNA Educational Starter Packet (ESP) – DVD Set & Book

For your convenience, supplements and tests kits can be found at the following websites:
www.holisticheal.com
www.longevityplus-rna.cm
www.longevityplus.com
www.testing4health.com

For more information regarding Dr. Yasko's autism protocol join the Parent Discussion Group at www.autismanswer.com.

Bibliography

A Relationship between Tylenol and Asthma. http://illness.altmedangel.com/asthma.htm. 2002; 21 May.

Aguilar, L., et al. FgF Modifies the Brain electrical activity. *Inst. Invest.* Neuroplast. Des. Cel. 1992; August.

Aravindakumar C., et al. Nitric oxide induces Zn+ release from metallothionein by destroying zinc-sulphur clusters without concomitant formation of S-nitrosothiol. *Biochem. J.* 1999; 344:253.

Aschner, et al. Methylmercury alters glutamate transport in astrocytes. *Neurochem Int.* 2000; 37:199.

Auger, Anthony P., et al. Mechanisms Of Steroid-Induced Brain Differentiation.http://www.tmin.ac.jp/sympo/98/mccarthy.html.2002;18 Apr

Atzori, M., et al. Dopamine-Acetycholine Interactions in the Modulation of glutamate Release. *Ann N.Y. Acad. Sci.* 2003; 1003:346

Aukrust P., et al. Decreased levels of total and reduced glutathione in CD4+ lymphocytes in common variable immunodeficiencies are associated with activation of the tumor necrosis factor system: possible immunopathogenic role of oxidative stress. *Blood.* 1995; 86:1383.

Babal, P., et al. Early Postnatal Glutamate Treatment Results in Altered Vascular Responsiveness. *Endocrine Regulations* 1998; 32: 33.

Bach, JF. Regulatory T Cells Under Scrutiny. *Nature Reviews Immunology*. 2003; 3:139.

Bartlett, John G., Neil R. Blacklow, and Sherwood L. Gorbach. *Infectious Diseases.* Philadelphia, PA: W.B. Saunders Company, 1998.

Bauer A., et al. Alpha-lipoic acid is an effective inhibitor of human immunodeficiency virus (HIV-1) replication. *Klinische Wochenschrift.* 1991; 69:722.

Bayliss, M. T., and M. S. Hickery. Interleukin- induced nitric oxide inhibits sulfation of glycosaminoglycan chains. *Biochim Biophys Acta* 1998; 1425: 282.

Bernard S., et al. Autism: A Unique Type of Mercury Poisoning. www.autism.com/ari/mercurylong.html 2000; June 27.

Biello, S. M., D. A. Golombek, and M. E. Harrington. Neuropeptide Y and glutamate block phase shifts in the suprachiasmatic nucleus in vitro. http://www.psy.gla.ac.uk/people/abstract.asp 1997; 25 June 2002

Binkley, Karen. Idiopathic Environmental Intolerance. *Journal of Allergy and Clinical Immunology* 2001;107: 887.

Blaylock, Russell. Interaction of Cytokines, Excitotoxins, and Reactive Nitrogen and Oxygen Species in Autism Spectrum Disorders. *JANA* 2003; 6 (4): 21.

Blaylock R. The Central Role of Excitotoxicity in Autism Spectrum Disorders. *JANA* 2003; 6(1): 10.

Blaylock, Russell L. Phytonutrients and Metabolic Stimulants as Protection Against Neurodegeneration and Excitotoxicity. *JANA* 2000; 2: 30.

Blaylock, Russell L. New Developments in the Prevention and Treatment of Neurodegenerative Diseases. *JANA* 2002; 5: 15-32.

Blaylock, Russell L. *Excitotoxins:The Taste that Kills*. Sante Fe, New Mexico: Health P, 1997.

Blue, M. E., et al. Postmortem Brain Abnormalities of the Glutamate Neurotransmitter System in Autism. *Neurology* 2001; 57: 1618.

Brinkworth R., et al. Inhibition of HIV-1 Proteinase by Non-peptide Carboxylates. *Biochem Biophy Res Commun* 1991; 176(1):241.

Brooks, D., et al. Molecular Characterization, Reactivation, and Depletion of Latent HIV. *Immunity* 2003; 19: 413.

Buckland, J. Tolerance or Immunity-Dendritic Cells Decide. *Nature Reviews Immunology*. 2003; 3(3): 182.

Campbell, J., M. A. Drake, and J. H. Isonhood. Impact of Salt and MSG on Survival of E. coli. http://ift.confex.com/ift/2002/techprogram/paper_13227.htm. 2002; 17 June

Carboxylation of glutamic acid. *The Merck Manual* (n.d.). 8 May 2002 http://www.merck.com/pubs/mmanual/figures/3fig2.htm.

Carlos, Juan. A New Look at Lipids in Nerves. *Nature Reviews*, 2004; 5.

Chelation of Mercury for the Treatment of Autism. 3 Mar. 2002 http://www.healing-arts.org/children/holmes.htm.

Clarkson T. The Three Modern Faces of Mercury. *Environmental Health Perspectives*. 2002; 110:11.

Cleary, P. P., Gary M. Dunny, and Larry L. McKay. Genetics *and Molecular Biology of Streptococci, Lactococci, and Enterococci.* Washington, DC: American Society for Microbiology, 1999.

Correll, et al. Use of Chemically Modified Nucleotides to Determine a 62 Nucleotide RNA Crystal Structure: A Survey of Phosphorothioates, Br, Pt, & Hg. *J Biomolecular Structure and Dynamics* 1997; 15(2):165

D'Adamo, Peter, and Catherine Whitney. *Eat Right 4 Your Type*. New York, NY: G.P. Putnam's Sons, 1996.

Daniels, Daniel H., Gregory W. Diachenko, and Frank L. Joe, Jr. Determination of Free Glutamic Acid in a Variety of Foods by High-performance Liquid Chromatography. *Food Additives and Contaminants* 1995;12 : 21-29.

Demirham I., Inhibition of Tat-mediated HIV-1-LTR Transactivation and Virus Replication by Sulfhydryl Compounds with Chelating Properties. *Anticancer Res.* 2000 ;20(4):2515.

Deth, Richard. Molecular *Origins of Human Attention, The Dopamine-Folate Connection*. Published by Kluwer.

Disease Statistics. http://www.msgtruth.org/disease.htm.9 June 2002

Drugs tested for Lou Gehrig's disease. *Science News* 2001; 160:23.

Dube, G. R., et al. Genetic enhancement of learning and memory in mice. *Nature* 1999; 401:63.

Edwards, C., et al. Auditory Midbrain Neurons That Count. *Nature Neuroscience* 2002; 5(10):934.

Effect Of Altered Expression Of The Cytoplasmic Copper-Zinc Superoxide Dismutase On Oxidative Stress Mediated Phenomena. http://lanfiles.williams.edu/~eadler/thesis/PJS1.html 1997; 25 June 2002.

Effects of Estrogens on Erythrocyte Antioxidant Superoxide Dismutase, Catalase and Glutathione Peroxidase Activities During Menstrual Cycle. *J Endocrinology* 2000; 167(3):447.

Eisenberg, J., et al. Haplotype Relative Risk Study of COMT and ADHD: Association of the High-enzyme Activity. *Am J. Med. Genet*. 1999; 88(5):497.

Evolutionary Discordance of Grains/Legumes in Diet. http://grains-legumes-b. html 18 June 2002.

Explorations of the New Frontier between Gut and Brain: A look at GAGs, CCK and Motilin. *1998 Durham Conference Psychobiology of Autism* http:// sunderland.ac.uk/autism.1998; 7 May 2002

Fleming, Richard and Tom Monte. *Stop Inflammation Now!* 2004

Florance, C. *Maverick Mind.* Published G.P. Putnam's Sons New York 2003.

Focus on Music. *Nature Neuroscience* 2003; 6(7) July.

Folkerth, Rebecca D., Preliminary Evidence: Herpesvirus Link to Mesial Temporal Lobe Epilepsy. *Jour. Watch Neur.* 2004; 6(3): 20.

From Inflammation and Autoimmunity to Nerve Regeneration and Protection. http://www.sciencedaily.com. 1999

Fujinami, R. and T. Sweeten. Letting Antibodies Get to Your Head. *Nature Medicine* 2003; 9(7):823.

Funseth E., et al. Effects of Coxsackievirus B3 Infection on Acute-phase Protein Metallothionein and on Cytochrome P-4501A1. *Sci Total Environ* 2002; 284(1):37.

Geiss G., et al. Global Impact of Influenza Virus on Cellular Pathways Is Mediated by Both Replication-Dependent and Independent Events. *J Virology* 2001; 75(9):4321.

Giacometti, T. Free and Bound Glutamate in Natural Products. Glutamic Acid:Advances in *Biochemistry and Physiology* 1979.

Glutamine: The Essential 'Non-Essential' Amino Acid. *Life Extension Magazine* 2002;199.

Gordon, G. EDTA and Chelation Therapy: History and Mechanisms of Action An Update. *Clinical Practice of Alternative Medicine* 2001; Volume 2(1):36-45.

Gordon, G. CHELATION DOCTOR, ASK YOURSELF "WHAT IF?" A Response to April Update by Elmer Cranton. *ACAM Journal* June 2003.

Gordon, G. and Joiner-Bey, H. *The Omega-3 Miracle.* 2004. Published by Freedom Press.

Gordon, G. and Yasko, A. Are RNA-Based Therapies the Biggest Breakthrough in NUTRITIONAL and Molecular Medicine? *Explore* 2004; 13(2):33-37.

Gould, S., et al. The Trojan Exosome Hypothesis. *PNAS* 2003; 100(19):10592.

Hans D., et al. Protection Against Glutamate-induced Cytotoxicity in C6 Glial Cells by Thiol Antioxidants. *Am J. Physiol* 1997; 273:1771.

Harder, B. Target: Celiac Disease. *Science News* . 2003; 163:392.

Hafez M., et al Susceptibility to Over Production of Cytokines in Acute Rheumatic Carditis and Their Role in the Pathogenesis. *J. Med. Sci.* 2002; 2(2):65.

Herbert, M. R. Localization of white matter volume increase in autism and developmental language disorder. *Annals of Neurology* 2004; 55:530.

Herman, J.G. and Baylin, S. Gene Silencing in Cancer in Association with Promoter Hypermethyation. *N. Engl J Med* 2003; 349:2042.

Hickery, M.S. and M.T. Bayliss. Interleukin- induced Nitric Oxide Inhibits Sulfation of Glycosaminoglycan Chains. *Biochim. Biophys. Acta.*1998;1425:282.

Hoffman, K., et al. A Murine Model for Neuropsychiatric Disorders Associated with Group A Streptococcal Infection. *J Neuroscience.* 2004; 24(7):1780.

Holden, Constance. Excited by Glutamate. *Science* 2003; 300: 1866.

Holden, Constance. Zapping Memory Craving Triggers Drug Craving. *Science* 2001;292:1039.

Hood, Ernie. RNAi: What's All the Noise About Gene Silencing? *Environmental Health Perspectives*. 2004; 112(4):A225-A229.

Ilback N., et al. Effects of Methylmercury on Cytokines, Inflammation, and Virus Clearance in a Common Infection. *Toxicology Letters* 1996; 89(1):19.

Jacoby, D. Virus-Induced Asthma Attacks. *J American Medical Association.* 2002. Vol 287:755.

Jacoby, M. Magnetic Fields and Unpolarized Light Have Hand in Chirality. *C & En.* 2000; 26:14.

Jezova, D., and D. Tokarev. Effect of Nitric Oxide Inhibition on Blood Pressure. *Physiol. Res.* 2000; 49:S87.

Jonata, P., et al. The Cortical Topography of Tonal Structures Underlying Western Music. *Science*. 2002; 298:2167.

Kasuya, E., et al. An increase in Glutamate Release in Female Rhesus Monkeys. *J. Neuroendocrinol.* 1999; 11:275.

Kasuya E., et al. A Role of GABA and Glutamate in Control of Puberty in Female. Rhesus Monkeys. *Endocrinology* 1999; 140(2):705.

Kegak, B. In Vitro Determaination of Specific Toxicity in Tetanus Vaccines. *Dev. Biol.* 2002; 111:27.

Kerblat, I. Tetanus Toxin L Chain is Processed by MHC Class I and Class II. *Immunology* 2000; 100:178.

Koland J. *Antineoplastic Agents I & II.* 2003; www.medicine.uiowa.edu/pharmacology/Lectures/ Lecturenotes/111/2004/

Lalli. G. Functional Characterization of Tentanus and Botulinum Neurotoxins Binding Domains. *J. Cell Sci.* 1999; 112:2715.

Larhammar, Dan. Neuropeptide Y and its Receptors: Physiology and Pharmacology. Molecular Properties, Ligand receptor Interactions, Roles in Appetite Regulation. 1 Dec. 2000; http://www.medfarm.neuro.uu.se/larhammar.html

Larson, H. Virtual Lab Conference. *Proceedings of the Fourth Session.* March 1-31 2003. www.afibbers.org/conference

Lee, T. H., et al. The role of Insulin in Interaction of Secretin and Cholecystokinin. *Pancreas* 12 (1996): 58.

Leo, M. A., and C. S. Lieber. Alcohol, Vitamin A, and Beta-carotene: Adverse Interactions. *American J. Clinical Nutrition* 1999; 69:1071.

Levitt J. Anxiety and Hypoglycemia What's the Connection? *Holistic Energy Magazine*. <www.hastingspress.co.uk/hypo/levitt.htm>.

Li, B., et al. Regulation of Muscarinic Acetylcholine Function in Acetylcholinesterase Knockout Mice. *Pharmacol. Biochem. Behav*. 2003; 74:977.

Li K., et al. Cellular Response to Conditional Expression of Hepatitis C Virus Core Protein in Huh7 Cultured Human Hepatoma Cells. *Hepatology* 2002; 35(5): 1237.

Lipids and Lou Gehrig's disease. *C&EN* / 26 August 2002: 30.

Marsicano, G., et ak. CB1 Cannabinoid Receptors and On-Demand Defense Against Excitotoxicity. *Science* 2003; 302:84.

Mattson, M.P., TerryAnn Perry, and Nigel H. Greig. Learning From the Gut. *Nature Medicine.* 2003; 9(9):1113.

McMichael J., et al. The Use of Low Dose Thimerosal for the Treatment of Herpesvirus Infections Non-*Linearity Conference Belle Umass Amherst.*

Mellman, I., and B. Winckler. Neuronal Polarity: Controlling the Sorting and Diffusion of Membrane Components. *Neuron.* 1999; 23:637. Milk Proteins As Potential Diet Aids. *Life Extension Magazine* 2002; June 22.

Mogadam, Michael. *Every Heart Attack Is Preventable*. 2001

Morales, J., et al. FgF Decreases seizure Frequency and Increases GABA Uptake. *Inst. Invest. Neuroplast. Des. Cel.*1992; August.

Munro, et al. High sensitivity of mouse neuronal cells to tetanus toxin requires a GPI-anchored protein. *Biochem Biophys Res Commun*. 2001; 289(2):623.

Nubrander, Biochemical Context and Clinical Use of Methylcobalamin. http://www.autisme-montreal.com/congress/2003/Neubrander.html.

NeuroGenesis Inc. The Stress Cycle. 18 June 2002 http://www.neurogenesis.cc/stresscycle.html.

Neuropeptide Y and its receptors: physiology and pharmacology. Molecular properties, ligand receptor interactions, roles in appetite regulation; 1997 http://arbl.cvmbs.colostate.edu/hbooks/pathphys/endocrine/bodyweight/npy.html.

Neuroprotection-Glutamate and Calpain Antagonism. 22 June 2002 http:// eardisorders.html.

Neuroscience and Music in Harmony. *New York Academy of Sciences Magazine.*2004; March.

Neyts J., et al. Effect of Iodo Deoxyuridine on Vaccinia Virus Infections in Mice. *Antimicrobial Agents and Chemotherapy* 2002; 46(9):2842.

NIAID Division of AIDS CHEMDB http://apps1.niaid.nih.gov/structsearch/default.htm. 2003; May 7.

Nicoll, Roger A., and Rachel I. Wilson. Endocannabinoid Signaling in the Brain. *Science*. 2002; 296 :678.

Nitrogen Metabolism and the Urea Cycle. 21 June 2002 http://216.23.../nitrogen-metabolism.html.

Nucleotides. www.rpi.edu/dept/bcbp/molbiochem/BiochSci/sbello/molbioch/nucleotides.htm.

Parslow, Tristram G., Daniel P. Stites, and Abba I. Terr. *Medical Immunology.* Stamford, CT: Appleton & Lange, 1997.

Poland, G., et al. The Association Between Measles Vaccine-induced Antibody Response and the HLA-DQA1 Alleles. *Vaccines 97,* page 229 Cold Spring Harbor Press.

Purcell, A.E., Jeon, O.H., Zimmerman, A.W., Blue, M.E, Pevsner, J. Postmortem Brain Abnormalities of the Glutamate Neurotransmitter System in Autism. *Neurology* 2001; 57(9): 1618-28.

Raloff, J. Little Vessels React to Magnetic Switch. *Science News* 2003; 163:270.

Scallet, A. C. Excitotoxic Mechanisms of Neurodegeneration in Transmissible Spongiform Encephalopathies. *Ann N Y Acad Sci.* 1997;Oct.

Schoonenberg, T. In the Blink of an Eye. Movement Disorders Team Report. www.hapsonline.org/public_http/Articles/EyeTroubles.pdf.

Seppa, Nathan. Glutamate Glut Linked to Multiple Sclerosis. *Science News* Jan. 8, 2000; Vol. 157, No. 2.

Seppa, Nathan. Chill Out: Mild Hypothermia Aids Heart Attack Recovery. *Science News* . 2002; 161(8):115.

Seppa, Nathan. Weak Appetite in Elderly Ties to Hormone. *Science News* 2001; 160:390.

Short Background of MSG. 9 June 2002.
South, James. Excitotoxins - the Ultimate Brainslayer. 23 June 2002 http:// ias-excitotoxins.htm.

Shnayerson, M. and Plotkin, M. *The Killers Within: The Deadly Rise of Drug-Resistant Bacteria*. 2002.

Spires, T., et al. Environmental Enrichment Rescues Protein Deficits. *Journal of Neuroscience.* 2004; 24(9):2270.

Spranger M., et al. Excess Glutamate in the Cerebrospinal Fluid in Bacterial Meningitis. *J. Neurol. Sci*. 1996; 143:126.

Steinman, D., Epstein, S. The Safe Shopper's Bible: A Consumer's Guide to Nontoxic Household Products.1995.Published by John Wiley & Sons.

Stokes, Ian. The NuTron Test. *Positive Health Magazine* 1998; 30:July.

Surtees, R., Leonard, J., and Austin, S. Association of Demyelination with Deficiency of Cerebrospinal Fluid S-adenosylmethionine in Inborn Errors of Methyl-transfer Pathway. *The Lancet* 1991; 338: 1550.

Taub, E., Ramey, S.L., DeLuca, S.C., Echols, K. Efficacy of Constrait induced (CI) Movement Therapy for Children With Cerebral Palsy. *Pediatrics*. 2004; 113(2):305.

Tamura G., et al. A Glutamine Transport Gene glnQ Is Required for Fibronectin Adherence and Virulence of Group B Streptococci. *Infection and Immunity*. 2002; 70(6):2877.

Tasker A., et al. Is Gastric Reflux a Cause of Otitis Media With Effusion in Children? *JAMA.* 2003; 289(11):1351.

Teplicky, et al. The Changes of Muscarinic , Beta adrenergic Receptors in Acetylcholinesterase Knockout Mice. Abstracts Department Physiology, Academy Sciences Czek Republic 2004.

Travers J, and E Helzner. Use of Dimercaptan Acids, Salts and Metabolites Thereof as Antiretroviral Treatment *US Patent* 1995.

Travis, John. Cancer Drugs may Thwart Huntington's. *Science News* 2001; 160(21): 332.

Travis, John. Drugs tested for Lou Gehrig's disease. *Science News* 2001; 160(23):362.

Travis, John. The Science of Secretin. *Science News.*2001;160:314.

Travis, John, Stimulating Clue hints How Lithium Works. *Science News Online* Feb. 14, 1998.

Tsakiris, S. Alanine Reverses the Inhibility Effect of Phenylalanine on Acetylchlinesterase Activity. *Z. Naturforsch.* 2002; 57c

Vaccines: The MMR Vaccine. 1 May 2002 http://vaccines-mmr.html.

Vaccine Scandal Revives Cancer Fear. *New Scientist.* 7 July 2004.

Vader, W., et al. The HLA-DQ2 Gene Dose Effect in Celiac Disease. *PNAS.* 2003;10:1073.

Vitamin K. *Life Extension Magazine*. 2000; 25 Mar. 2002 http://www.lef.org/magazine/mag2000/feb00-report.html.

Vojdani, A., et al. Antibodies to Neuron-specific Antigens in Children with Autism. *J of Neuroimmunology.* 2003;129 (1): 168.

Waly, M., et al. Activation of Methione Synthase by Insulin-like Growth Factor-1 and Dopamine. *Molecular Psychiatry*. 2004; 1-13.

Ward D., et al. Direct Mercuration of Nucleotides and Polynucleotides. *Biochemistry* 1975; 14(11):2447.

Weinstein, Y., et al. Sex Associated Differences in the Regulation of Immune Responses Controlled by the MHC of the Mouse. *J of Immunology.* 1984; 132:656.

Wells and Wilkins, Clostridia http://gsbs.utmb.edu/microbook/ch018.htm. What are Hydrolyzed Proteins. 22 June 2002 <http://msg.html>.

What Came Before DNA? *Discover*. June 2004.

Williams D. Muck Up a Leaky Gut. *Alternatives*. 2003; February:156.

Williams D. Magnetically Attractive Healing. *Alternatives*. 2004; March:65.

Woodbury, D. J., Miller, C. Nystatin induced liposome fusion: A versatile approach to ion channel reconstitution into planar bilayers. *Biophys. J.* 1990; 58:833.

Wunderlich V, and G. Sydow. Disintegration of Retroviruses by Chelating Agents. *Archives of Virology* 1982; 73:171.

Yasko A. The Role of Excitotoxins in Autistic Type Behavior. www.holistichealth.com. 2002; June 16.

Yasko A. Autism: A Twisted Tale of Virus and Thimerosal. www.holistichealth.com. 2003; May 31.

Yu, A J and Dayan, P. Acetylcholine, Norepinephrine, and Spatial Attention. Elsevier computer Science Preprint Server, 2003.

Zhu, B. COMT Mediated Methylation Metabolism of Endogenous Bioactive Catehols. *Current Drug Metabolism.* 2002; 3(3): 321.

Zhu H., et al. Cu (2+) Suppresses GABA (A) Receptor-Mediated Responses in Rat Sacral Dorsal Commissural Neurons. *Neurosignals* 2002; 11(6): 322.

Zubieta, J., et al. COMT Val 158met Genotype Affects u-Opioid Neurotransmitter Responses to a Pain Stressor. *Science.* 2003; 299(5610): 1240.

Zweiger, Gary. *Transducing the Genome*. 2001.

Sample Detoxification Data

By the grace of God, I met Amy in November 2004 and became her client immediately thereafter. My daughter Madison was 2 and ½ years old and had been diagnosed with PDD. At this time Madison had very poor gross motor skills (she did not walk until she was over 2 years old); she had low energy, and poor receptive learning abilities. For the most part she was way behind her peers on all levels. Amy evaluated all of her medical records and correctly diagnosed Madison as someone who had a high metal load that was affecting her nervous and muscular systems. She told us that she would first correct the gross motor and physical issues by eliminating the metals from her body and reversing the mitochondria blockage. Next she would attack the bowel issues and lastly we would see vast improvement in her ability to process (her receptive learning skills).

Today, almost 15 months later, Madison is a new child. Her gross motor skills are now at age appropriate levels. She has normal bowels and she can answer questions and process verbal requests with little or no delay. She will be attending a regular school in the fall. In other words, thanks to Amy, our daughter is healed and her prospects of living a normal life are excellent. I thank God for the work Amy is doing to heal kids on the Autistic spectrum.

JM, Texas

URINE TOXIC METALS

DOCTOR'S DATA INC

LAB#:
PATIENT:
SEX: Male
AGE: 4

CLIENT#: 27080
DOCTOR: Amy Yasko, ND
Holistic Health
Po Box 309
Bethel, ME 04217

POTENTIALLY TOXIC METALS

METALS	RESULT µg/g CREAT	REFERENCE RANGE	WITHIN REFERENCE RANGE	ELEVATED	VERY ELEVATED
Aluminum	< dl	< 35			
Antimony	< dl	< 5			
Arsenic	92	< 100			
Beryllium	< dl	< 0.5			
Bismuth	< dl	< 30			
Cadmium	< dl	< 2			
Lead	< dl	< 15			
Mercury	15	< 3			
Nickel	< dl	< 12			
Platinum	< dl	< 2			
Thallium	2.3	< 14			
Thorium	< dl	< 12			
Tin	< dl	< 6			
Tungsten	< dl	< 23			
Uranium	< dl	< 1			

CREATININE

	RESULT mg/dL	REFERENCE RANGE	2SD LOW	1SD LOW	MEAN	1SD HIGH	2SD HIGH
Creatinine	13	21- 76					

SPECIMEN DATA

Comments:

Date Collected:	8/1/2003	Method:	ICP-MS	Collection Period:	Random
Date Received:	8/4/2003	<dl:	less than detection limit	Volume:	
Date Completed:	8/5/2003	Provoking Agent:		Provocation:	PRE PROVOCATIVE

URINE TOXIC METALS

DOCTOR'S DATA INC

LAB#:
PATIENT:
SEX: Male
AGE: 4

CLIENT#: 27080
DOCTOR: Amy Yasko, ND
Holistic Health
Po Box 309
Bethel, ME 04217

POTENTIALLY TOXIC METALS

METALS	RESULT µg/g CREAT	REFERENCE RANGE	WITHIN REFERENCE RANGE	ELEVATED	VERY ELEVATED
Aluminum	120	< 35			
Antimony	< dl	< 5			
Arsenic	78	< 100			
Beryllium	< dl	< 0.5			
Bismuth	< dl	< 30			
Cadmium	0.7	< 2			
Lead	3.8	< 15			
Mercury	12	< 3			
Nickel	5.2	< 12			
Platinum	< dl	< 2			
Thallium	2.2	< 14			
Thorium	0.2	< 12			
Tin	2.8	< 6			
Tungsten	0.3	< 23			
Uranium	< dl	< 1			

CREATININE

	RESULT mg/dL	REFERENCE RANGE	2SD LOW	1SD LOW	MEAN	1SD HIGH	2SD HIGH
Creatinine	26	21- 76					

SPECIMEN DATA

Comments:					
Date Collected:	8/5/2003	Method:	ICP-MS	Collection Period:	Random
Date Received:	8/7/2003	<dl:	less than detection limit	Volume:	
Date Completed:	8/15/2003	Provoking Agent:		Provocation:	POST

URINE TOXIC METALS

DOCTOR'S DATA INC

LAB#:
PATIENT:
SEX: Male
AGE: 2

CLIENT#: 27080
DOCTOR: Amy Yasko, ND
Holistic Health
Po Box 309
Bethel, ME 04217

POTENTIALLY TOXIC METALS

METALS	RESULT µg/g CREAT	REFERENCE RANGE	WITHIN REFERENCE RANGE	ELEVATED	VERY ELEVATED
Aluminum	2700	< 100			
Antimony	0.8	< 2			
Arsenic	130	< 200			
Beryllium	< dl	< 0.6			
Bismuth	< dl	< 20			
Cadmium	1.8	< 3			
Lead	0.4	< 5			
Mercury	< dl	< 5			
Nickel	11	< 20			
Platinum	< dl	< 1			
Thallium	0.4	< 1.1			
Thorium	0.4	< 1			
Tin	9.2	< 20			
Tungsten	0.6	< 2			
Uranium	< dl	< 0.3			

CREATININE

	RESULT mg/dL	REFERENCE RANGE	2SD LOW	1SD LOW	MEAN	1SD HIGH	2SD HIGH
Creatinine	48	15- 120					

SPECIMEN DATA

Comments:					
Date Collected:	10/29/2005	Method:	ICP-MS	Collection Period:	timed: 5 hours
Date Received:	11/1/2005	<dl:	less than detection limit	Volume:	
Date Completed:	11/6/2005	Provoking Agent:		Provocation:	

Toxic metals are reported as µg/g creatinine to account for urine dilution variations. **Reference ranges are representative of a healthy population under non-challenge or non-provoked conditions.** No safe reference levels for toxic metals have been established.

V10.00

URINE TOXIC METALS

DOCTOR'S DATA INC

LAB#:
PATIENT:
SEX: Female
AGE: 7

CLIENT#: 27080
DOCTOR: Amy Yasko, ND
Holistic Health
Po Box 309
Bethel, ME 04217

POTENTIALLY TOXIC METALS

METALS	RESULT µg/g CREAT	REFERENCE RANGE	WITHIN REFERENCE RANGE	ELEVATED	VERY ELEVATED
Aluminum	560	< 60			
Antimony	1.7	< 1.5			
Arsenic	23	< 130			
Beryllium	< dl	< 0.6			
Bismuth	3.3	< 20			
Cadmium	1.7	< 2			
Lead	0.4	< 5			
Mercury	2.8	< 5			
Nickel	5.8	< 15			
Platinum	< dl	< 1			
Thallium	< dl	< 1.1			
Thorium	< dl	< 0.5			
Tin	65	< 15			
Tungsten	0.5	< 1.5			
Uranium	< dl	< 0.2			

CREATININE

	RESULT mg/dL	REFERENCE RANGE	2SD LOW	1SD LOW	MEAN	1SD HIGH	2SD HIGH
Creatinine	48	25- 180					

SPECIMEN DATA

Comments:

Date Collected:	12/15/2005	Method:	ICP-MS	Collection Period:	Random
Date Received:	12/16/2005	<dl:	less than detection limit	Volume:	
Date Completed:	12/20/2005	Provoking Agent:		Provocation:	

Toxic metals are reported as µg/g creatinine to account for urine dilution variations. **Reference ranges are representative of a healthy population under non-challenge or non-provoked conditions.** No safe reference levels for toxic metals have been established.

V10.00

URINE TOXIC METALS

DOCTOR'S DATA INC

LAB#:
PATIENT:
SEX: Male
AGE: 11

CLIENT#: 27080
DOCTOR: Amy Yasko, ND
Holistic Health
Po Box 309
Bethel, ME 04217

POTENTIALLY TOXIC METALS

METALS	RESULT µg/g CREAT	REFERENCE RANGE	WITHIN REFERENCE RANGE	ELEVATED	VERY ELEVATED
Aluminum	1020	< 60			
Antimony	0.3	< 1.5			
Arsenic	47	< 130			
Beryllium	< dl	< 0.6			
Bismuth	< dl	< 20			
Cadmium	1	< 2			
Lead	< dl	< 5			
Mercury	1.8	< 5			
Nickel	8.3	< 15			
Platinum	< dl	< 1			
Thallium	0.4	< 1.1			
Thorium	< dl	< 0.5			
Tin	1.2	< 15			
Tungsten	0.3	< 1.5			
Uranium	< dl	< 0.2			

CREATININE

	RESULT mg/dL	REFERENCE RANGE	2SD LOW	1SD LOW	MEAN	1SD HIGH	2SD HIGH
Creatinine	30	25- 180					

SPECIMEN DATA

Comments:

Date Collected:	10/23/2005	Method:	ICP-MS	Collection Period:	Random
Date Received:	10/26/2005	<dl:	less than detection limit	Volume:	
Date Completed:	10/31/2005	Provoking Agent:		Provocation:	

Toxic metals are reported as µg/g creatinine to account for urine dilution variations. **Reference ranges are representative of a healthy population under non-challenge or non-provoked conditions.** No safe reference levels for toxic metals have been established. V10.00

URINE TOXIC METALS

DOCTOR'S DATA INC

LAB#:
PATIENT:
SEX: Male
AGE: 5

CLIENT#: 27080
DOCTOR: Amy Yasko, ND
Holistic Health
Po Box 309
Bethel, ME 04217

POTENTIALLY TOXIC METALS

METALS	RESULT µg/g CREAT	REFERENCE RANGE	WITHIN REFERENCE RANGE	ELEVATED	VERY ELEVATED
Aluminum	< dl	< 60			
Antimony	< dl	< 1.5			
Arsenic	31	< 130			
Beryllium	< dl	< 0.6			
Bismuth	< dl	< 20			
Cadmium	2	< 2			
Lead	< dl	< 5			
Mercury	46	< 5			
Nickel	< dl	< 15			
Platinum	< dl	< 1			
Thallium	< dl	< 1.1			
Thorium	< dl	< 0.5			
Tin	< dl	< 15			
Tungsten	< dl	< 1.5			
Uranium	< dl	< 0.2			

CREATININE

	RESULT mg/dL	REFERENCE RANGE	2SD LOW	1SD LOW	MEAN	1SD HIGH	2SD HIGH
Creatinine	6.9	25- 180					

SPECIMEN DATA

Comments:

Date Collected:	12/7/2005	Method:	ICP-MS	Collection Period:	Random
Date Received:	12/9/2005	<dl:	less than detection limit	Volume:	
Date Completed:	12/12/2005	Provoking Agent:		Provocation:	

Toxic metals are reported as µg/g creatinine to account for urine dilution variations. **Reference ranges are representative of a healthy population under non-challenge or non-provoked conditions.** No safe reference levels for toxic metals have been established.

V10.00

URINE TOXIC METALS

DOCTOR'S DATA INC

LAB#:
PATIENT:
SEX: Female
AGE: 5

CLIENT#: 27080
DOCTOR: Amy Yasko, ND
Holistic Health
Po Box 309
Bethel, ME 04217

POTENTIALLY TOXIC METALS

METALS	RESULT µg/g CREAT	REFERENCE RANGE	WITHIN REFERENCE RANGE	ELEVATED	VERY ELEVATED
Aluminum	< dl	< 60			
Antimony	7.3	< 1.5			
Arsenic	180	< 130			
Beryllium	< dl	< 0.6			
Bismuth	< dl	< 20			
Cadmium	1.6	< 2			
Lead	13	< 5			
Mercury	22	< 5			
Nickel	< dl	< 15			
Platinum	1	< 1			
Thallium	1.1	< 1.1			
Thorium	< dl	< 0.5			
Tin	< dl	< 15			
Tungsten	15	< 1.5			
Uranium	< dl	< 0.2			

CREATININE

	RESULT mg/dL	REFERENCE RANGE	2SD LOW	1SD LOW	MEAN	1SD HIGH	2SD HIGH
Creatinine	6.3	25- 180					

SPECIMEN DATA

Comments:

Date Collected:	11/23/2005	Method:	ICP-MS	Collection Period:	Random
Date Received:	12/1/2005	<dl:	less than detection limit	Volume:	
Date Completed:	12/7/2005	Provoking Agent:		Provocation:	

Toxic metals are reported as µg/g creatinine to account for urine dilution variations. **Reference ranges are representative of a healthy population under non-challenge or non-provoked conditions.** No safe reference levels for toxic metals have been established. V10.00

URINE TOXIC METALS

DOCTOR'S DATA Inc

LAB#:
PATIENT:
SEX: Female
AGE: 3

CLIENT#: 27080
DOCTOR: Amy Yasko, ND
Holistic Health
Po Box 309
Bethel, ME 04217

POTENTIALLY TOXIC METALS

METALS	RESULT µg/g CREAT	REFERENCE RANGE	WITHIN REFERENCE RANGE	ELEVATED	VERY ELEVATED
Aluminum	2390	< 100			
Antimony	12	< 2			
Arsenic	62	< 200			
Beryllium	< dl	< 0.6			
Bismuth	24	< 20			
Cadmium	3.4	< 3			
Lead	80	< 5			
Mercury	7	< 5			
Nickel	210	< 20			
Platinum	< dl	< 1			
Thallium	0.4	< 1.1			
Thorium	0.5	< 1			
Tin	95	< 20			
Tungsten	4.8	< 2			
Uranium	7.8	< 0.3			

CREATININE

	RESULT mg/dL	REFERENCE RANGE	2SD LOW	1SD LOW	MEAN	1SD HIGH	2SD HIGH
Creatinine	14	15- 120					

SPECIMEN DATA

Comments: insufficient sample to recheck results

Date Collected:	7/13/2005	Method:	ICP-MS	Collection Period:	Random
Date Received:	7/15/2005	<dl:	less than detection limit	Volume:	
Date Completed:	7/21/2005	Provoking Agent:		Provocation:	

Toxic metals are reported as µg/g creatinine to account for urine dilution variations. **Reference ranges are representative of a healthy population under non-challenge or non-provoked conditions.** No safe reference levels for toxic metals have been established. V10.00

URINE TOXIC METALS

DOCTOR'S DATA

LAB#:
PATIENT:
SEX: Male
AGE: 11

CLIENT#: 27080
DOCTOR: Amy Yasko, ND
Holistic Health
Po Box 309
Bethel, ME 04217

POTENTIALLY TOXIC METALS

METALS	RESULT µg/g CREAT	REFERENCE RANGE	WITHIN REFERENCE RANGE	ELEVATED	VERY ELEVATED
Aluminum	< dl	< 60			
Antimony	< dl	< 1.5			
Arsenic	77	< 130			
Beryllium	< dl	< 0.6			
Bismuth	< dl	< 20			
Cadmium	1.6	< 2			
Lead	43	< 5			
Mercury	2.6	< 5			
Nickel	3.6	< 15			
Platinum	< dl	< 1			
Thallium	< dl	< 1.1			
Thorium	< dl	< 0.5			
Tin	< dl	< 15			
Tungsten	< dl	< 1.5			
Uranium	< dl	< 0.2			

CREATININE

	RESULT mg/dL	REFERENCE RANGE	2SD LOW	1SD LOW	MEAN	1SD HIGH	2SD HIGH
Creatinine	14	25- 180					

SPECIMEN DATA

Comments:

Date Collected:	12/26/2005	Method:	ICP-MS	Collection Period:	Random
Date Received:	12/28/2005	<dl:	less than detection limit	Volume:	
Date Completed:	12/29/2005	Provoking Agent:		Provocation:	

Toxic metals are reported as µg/g creatinine to account for urine dilution variations. **Reference ranges are representative of a healthy population under non-challenge or non-provoked conditions.** No safe reference levels for toxic metals have been established.

V10.00

URINE TOXIC METALS

DOCTOR'S DATA INC.

LAB#:
PATIENT:
SEX: Male
AGE: 4

CLIENT#: 27080
DOCTOR: Amy Yasko, ND
Holistic Health
Po Box 309
Bethel, ME 04217

POTENTIALLY TOXIC METALS

METALS	RESULT µg/g CREAT	REFERENCE RANGE	WITHIN REFERENCE RANGE	ELEVATED	VERY ELEVATED
Aluminum	< dl	< 35			
Antimony	0.5	< 5			
Arsenic	91	< 100			
Beryllium	< dl	< 0.5			
Bismuth	< dl	< 30			
Cadmium	1.7	< 2			
Lead	< dl	< 15			
Mercury	19	< 3			
Nickel	4.4	< 12			
Platinum	< dl	< 2			
Thallium	0.4	< 14			
Thorium	< dl	< 12			
Tin	1.8	< 6			
Tungsten	5.1	< 23			
Uranium	< dl	< 1			

CREATININE

	RESULT mg/dL	REFERENCE RANGE	2SD LOW	1SD LOW	MEAN	1SD HIGH	2SD HIGH
Creatinine	14	21- 76					

SPECIMEN DATA

Comments:					
Date Collected:	9/13/2003	Method:	ICP-MS	Collection Period:	Random
Date Received:	9/15/2003	<dl:	less than detection limit	Volume:	
Date Completed:	9/16/2003	Provoking Agent:		Provocation:	

URINE TOXIC METALS

DOCTOR'S DATA INC

LAB#:
PATIENT:
SEX: Male
AGE: 5

CLIENT#: 27080
DOCTOR: Amy Yasko, ND
Holistic Health
Po Box 309
Bethel, ME 04217

POTENTIALLY TOXIC METALS

METALS	RESULT µg/g CREAT	REFERENCE RANGE	WITHIN REFERENCE RANGE	ELEVATED	VERY ELEVATED
Aluminum	38	< 35			
Antimony	< dl	< 5			
Arsenic	34	< 100			
Beryllium	< dl	< 0.5			
Bismuth	< dl	< 30			
Cadmium	< dl	< 2			
Lead	1.3	< 15			
Mercury	13	< 3			
Nickel	4.4	< 12			
Platinum	< dl	< 2			
Thallium	0.8	< 14			
Thorium	< dl	< 12			
Tin	2.1	< 6			
Tungsten	< dl	< 23			
Uranium	< dl	< 1			

CREATININE

	RESULT mg/dL	REFERENCE RANGE	2SD LOW	1SD LOW	MEAN	1SD HIGH	2SD HIGH
Creatinine	25	40- 142					

SPECIMEN DATA

Comments:

Date Collected:	8/20/2003	Method:	ICP-MS	Collection Period:	Random
Date Received:	8/22/2003	<dl:	less than detection limit	Volume:	
Date Completed:	8/23/2003	Provoking Agent:		Provocation:	

URINE TOXIC METALS

LAB#: PATIENT: SEX: Male AGE: 3	CLIENT#: 27080 DOCTOR: Amy Yasko, ND Holistic Health Po Box 309 Bethel, ME 04217

POTENTIALLY TOXIC METALS

METALS	RESULT µg/g CREAT	REFERENCE RANGE	WITHIN REFERENCE RANGE	ELEVATED	VERY ELEVATED
Aluminum	40	< 35			
Antimony	0.2	< 5			
Arsenic	23	< 100			
Beryllium	< dl	< 0.5			
Bismuth	< dl	< 30			
Cadmium	0.7	< 2			
Lead	16	< 15			
Mercury	1.7	< 3			
Nickel	2.2	< 12			
Platinum	< dl	< 2			
Thallium	0.8	< 14			
Thorium	< dl	< 12			
Tin	97	< 6			
Tungsten	0.2	< 23			
Uranium	< dl	< 1			

CREATININE

	RESULT mg/dL	REFERENCE RANGE	2SD LOW	1SD LOW	MEAN	1SD HIGH	2SD HIGH
Creatinine	45	21- 76					

SPECIMEN DATA

Comments:					
Date Collected:	9/17/2003	Method:	ICP-MS	Collection Period:	Random
Date Received:	9/19/2003	<dl:	less than detection limit	Volume:	
Date Completed:	9/20/2003	Provoking Agent:		Provocation:	

URINE TOXIC METALS

DOCTOR'S DATA INC

LAB#:
PATIENT:
SEX: Male
AGE: 3

CLIENT#: 27080
DOCTOR: Amy Yasko, ND
Holistic Health
Po Box 309
Bethel, ME 04217

POTENTIALLY TOXIC METALS

METALS	RESULT µg/g CREAT	REFERENCE RANGE	WITHIN REFERENCE RANGE	ELEVATED	VERY ELEVATED
Aluminum	82	< 35			
Antimony	0.3	< 5			
Arsenic	14	< 100			
Beryllium	< dl	< 0.5			
Bismuth	0.3	< 30			
Cadmium	5.5	< 2			
Lead	5.4	< 15			
Mercury	< dl	< 3			
Nickel	5.3	< 12			
Platinum	< dl	< 2			
Thallium	0.5	< 14			
Thorium	0.07	< 12			
Tin	140	< 6			
Tungsten	0.1	< 23			
Uranium	0.1	< 1			

CREATININE

	RESULT mg/dL	REFERENCE RANGE	2SD LOW	1SD LOW	MEAN	1SD HIGH	2SD HIGH
Creatinine	37	21- 76					

SPECIMEN DATA

Comments: results checked
Date Collected: 9/19/2003
Date Received: 9/22/2003
Date Completed: 9/24/2003

Method: ICP-MS
<dl: less than detection limit
Provoking Agent:

Collection Period: Random
Volume:
Provocation:

URINE TOXIC METALS

DOCTOR'S DATA INC

LAB#:
PATIENT:
SEX: Male
AGE: 7

CLIENT#: 27080
DOCTOR: Amy Yasko, ND
Holistic Health
Po Box 309
Bethel, ME 04217

POTENTIALLY TOXIC METALS

METALS	RESULT µg/g CREAT	REFERENCE RANGE	WITHIN REFERENCE RANGE	ELEVATED	VERY ELEVATED
Aluminum	< dl	< 60			
Antimony	< dl	< 1.5			
Arsenic	54	< 130			
Beryllium	< dl	< 0.6			
Bismuth	< dl	< 20			
Cadmium	0.7	< 2			
Lead	< dl	< 18			
Mercury	1.1	< 5			
Nickel	4.8	< 15			
Platinum	< dl	< 1			
Thallium	< dl	< 1			
Thorium	< dl	< 0.5			
Tin	< dl	< 15			
Tungsten	5.7	< 1.5			
Uranium	< dl	< 0.2			

CREATININE

	RESULT mg/dL	REFERENCE RANGE	2SD LOW	1SD LOW	MEAN	1SD HIGH	2SD HIGH
Creatinine	55	40- 142					

SPECIMEN DATA

Comments:
Date Collected: 10/14/2003
Date Received: 10/16/2003
Date Completed: 10/23/2003

Method: ICP-MS
<dl: less than detection limit
Provoking Agent:

Collection Period: timed: 2 hours
Volume:
Provocation: POST PROVOCATIVE

URINE TOXIC METALS

DOCTOR'S DATA INC

LAB#:
PATIENT:
SEX: Male
AGE: 4

CLIENT#: 27080
DOCTOR: Amy Yasko, ND
Holistic Health
Po Box 309
Bethel, ME 04217

POTENTIALLY TOXIC METALS

METALS	RESULT µg/g CREAT	REFERENCE RANGE	WITHIN REFERENCE RANGE	ELEVATED	VERY ELEVATED
Aluminum	< dl	< 35			
Antimony	< dl	< 5			
Arsenic	38	< 100			
Beryllium	< dl	< 0.5			
Bismuth	< dl	< 30			
Cadmium	< dl	< 2			
Lead	33	< 15			
Mercury	24	< 3			
Nickel	< dl	< 12			
Platinum	< dl	< 2			
Thallium	< dl	< 14			
Thorium	< dl	< 12			
Tin	< dl	< 6			
Tungsten	< dl	< 23			
Uranium	< dl	< 1			

CREATININE

	RESULT mg/dL	REFERENCE RANGE	2SD LOW	1SD LOW	MEAN	1SD HIGH	2SD HIGH
Creatinine	4.6	21- 76					

SPECIMEN DATA

Comments:

Date Collected:	8/21/2003	Method:	ICP-MS	Collection Period:	Random
Date Received:	8/22/2003	<dl:	less than detection limit	Volume:	
Date Completed:	8/23/2003	Provoking Agent:		Provocation:	PRE PROVOCATIVE

URINE TOXIC METALS

DOCTOR'S DATA INC.

LAB#:
PATIENT:
SEX: Male
AGE: 3

CLIENT#: 27080
DOCTOR: Amy Yasko, ND
Holistic Health
Po Box 309
Bethel, ME 04217

POTENTIALLY TOXIC METALS

METALS	RESULT µg/g CREAT	REFERENCE RANGE	WITHIN REFERENCE RANGE	ELEVATED	VERY ELEVATED
Aluminum	< dl	< 100			
Antimony	< dl	< 2			
Arsenic	140	< 200			
Beryllium	< dl	< 0.6			
Bismuth	< dl	< 20			
Cadmium	7.9	< 3			
Lead	0.4	< 20			
Mercury	1.5	< 5			
Nickel	7.5	< 20			
Platinum	< dl	< 1			
Thallium	0.2	< 1.1			
Thorium	< dl	< 1			
Tin	11	< 20			
Tungsten	0.6	< 2			
Uranium	< dl	< 0.3			

CREATININE

	RESULT mg/dL	REFERENCE RANGE	2SD LOW	1SD LOW	MEAN	1SD HIGH	2SD HIGH
Creatinine	45	21- 76					

SPECIMEN DATA

Comments:

Date Collected:	3/30/2004	Method:	ICP-MS	Collection Period:	Random
Date Received:	4/1/2004	<dl:	less than detection limit	Volume:	
Date Completed:	4/2/2004	Provoking Agent:		Provocation:	

URINE TOXIC METALS

DOCTOR'S DATA INC

LAB#:
PATIENT:
SEX: Male
AGE: 4

CLIENT#: 27080
DOCTOR: Amy Yasko, ND
Holistic Health
Po Box 309
Bethel, ME 04217

POTENTIALLY TOXIC METALS

METALS	RESULT µg/g CREAT	REFERENCE RANGE	WITHIN REFERENCE RANGE	ELEVATED	VERY ELEVATED
Aluminum	180	< 35			
Antimony	0.5	< 5			
Arsenic	72	< 100			
Beryllium	< dl	< 0.5			
Bismuth	< dl	< 30			
Cadmium	0.6	< 2			
Lead	< dl	< 15			
Mercury	10	< 3			
Nickel	2.6	< 12			
Platinum	< dl	< 2			
Thallium	3.2	< 14			
Thorium	< dl	< 12			
Tin	1.2	< 6			
Tungsten	3.5	< 23			
Uranium	< dl	< 1			

CREATININE

	RESULT mg/dL	REFERENCE RANGE	2SD LOW	1SD LOW	MEAN	1SD HIGH	2SD HIGH
Creatinine	14	21- 76					

SPECIMEN DATA

Comments:

Date Collected:	7/24/2003	Method:	ICP-MS	Collection Period:	Random
Date Received:	7/25/2003	<dl:	less than detection limit	Volume:	
Date Completed:	7/29/2003	Provoking Agent:		Provocation:	PRE PROVOCATIVE

URINE TOXIC METALS

DOCTOR'S DATA INC

LAB#:
PATIENT:
SEX: Male
AGE: 8

CLIENT#: 27080
DOCTOR: Amy Yasko, ND
Holistic Health
Po Box 309
Bethel, ME 04217

POTENTIALLY TOXIC METALS

METALS	RESULT µg/g CREAT	REFERENCE RANGE	WITHIN REFERENCE RANGE	ELEVATED	VERY ELEVATED
Aluminum	< dl	< 60			
Antimony	< dl	< 1.5			
Arsenic	37	< 130			
Beryllium	< dl	< 0.6			
Bismuth	< dl	< 20			
Cadmium	< dl	< 2			
Lead	< dl	< 18			
Mercury	12	< 5			
Nickel	< dl	< 15			
Platinum	< dl	< 1			
Thallium	0.5	< 1.1			
Thorium	< dl	< 0.5			
Tin	< dl	< 15			
Tungsten	< dl	< 1.5			
Uranium	< dl	< 0.2			

CREATININE

	RESULT mg/dL	REFERENCE RANGE	2SD LOW	1SD LOW	MEAN	1SD HIGH	2SD HIGH
Creatinine	15	40- 142					

SPECIMEN DATA

Comments:					
Date Collected:	2/24/2004	Method:	ICP-MS	Collection Period:	Random
Date Received:	2/26/2004	<dl:	less than detection limit	Volume:	
Date Completed:	2/28/2004	Provoking Agent:		Provocation:	POST PROVOCATIVF

URINE TOXIC METALS

DOCTOR'S DATA INC

LAB#:
PATIENT:
SEX: Male
AGE: 6

CLIENT#: 27080
DOCTOR: Amy Yasko, ND
Holistic Health
Po Box 309
Bethel, ME 04217

POTENTIALLY TOXIC METALS

METALS	RESULT µg/g CREAT	REFERENCE RANGE	WITHIN REFERENCE RANGE	ELEVATED	VERY ELEVATED
Aluminum	< dl	< 60			
Antimony	< dl	< 1.5			
Arsenic	47	< 130			
Beryllium	< dl	< 0.6			
Bismuth	< dl	< 20			
Cadmium	0.8	< 2			
Lead	< dl	< 18			
Mercury	11	< 5			
Nickel	< dl	< 15			
Platinum	< dl	< 1			
Thallium	1.2	< 1.1			
Thorium	< dl	< 0.5			
Tin	< dl	< 15			
Tungsten	< dl	< 1.5			
Uranium	< dl	< 0.2			

CREATININE

	RESULT mg/dL	REFERENCE RANGE	2SD LOW	1SD LOW	MEAN	1SD HIGH	2SD HIGH
Creatinine	11	40- 142					

SPECIMEN DATA

Comments:

Date Collected:	3/18/2004	Method:	ICP-MS	Collection Period:	Random
Date Received:	3/24/2004	<dl:	less than detection limit	Volume:	
Date Completed:	3/25/2004	Provoking Agent:		Provocation:	

URINE TOXIC METALS

DOCTOR'S DATA INC

LAB#:
PATIENT:
SEX: Male
AGE: 8

CLIENT#: 27080
DOCTOR: Amy Yasko, ND
Holistic Health
Po Box 309
Bethel, ME 04217

POTENTIALLY TOXIC METALS

METALS	RESULT µg/g CREAT	REFERENCE RANGE	WITHIN REFERENCE RANGE	ELEVATED	VERY ELEVATED
Aluminum	< dl	< 60			
Antimony	< dl	< 1.5			
Arsenic	17	< 130			
Beryllium	< dl	< 0.6			
Bismuth	< dl	< 20			
Cadmium	< dl	< 2			
Lead	2.1	< 18			
Mercury	12	< 5			
Nickel	< dl	< 15			
Platinum	< dl	< 1			
Thallium	< dl	< 1.1			
Thorium	< dl	< 0.5			
Tin	< dl	< 15			
Tungsten	0.7	< 1.5			
Uranium	< dl	< 0.2			

CREATININE

	RESULT mg/dL	REFERENCE RANGE	2SD LOW	1SD LOW	MEAN	1SD HIGH	2SD HIGH
Creatinine	8.2	40- 142					

SPECIMEN DATA

Comments:

Date Collected: 11/18/2003
Date Received: 11/19/2003
Date Completed: 11/20/2003

Method: ICP-MS
<dl: less than detection limit
Provoking Agent:

Collection Period: Random
Volume:
Provocation: PRE PROVOCATIVE

URINE TOXIC METALS

DOCTOR'S DATA INC

LAB#:
PATIENT:
SEX: Male
AGE: 7

CLIENT#: 27080
DOCTOR: Amy Yasko, ND
Holistic Health
Po Box 309
Bethel, ME 04217

POTENTIALLY TOXIC METALS

METALS	RESULT µg/g CREAT	REFERENCE RANGE	WITHIN REFERENCE RANGE	ELEVATED	VERY ELEVATED
Aluminum	< dl	< 60			
Antimony	< dl	< 1.5			
Arsenic	76	< 130			
Beryllium	< dl	< 0.6			
Bismuth	< dl	< 20			
Cadmium	0.4	< 2			
Lead	< dl	< 18			
Mercury	1.4	< 5			
Nickel	< dl	< 15			
Platinum	< dl	< 1			
Thallium	1.1	< 1.1			
Thorium	< dl	< 0.5			
Tin	< dl	< 15			
Tungsten	8.8	< 1.5			
Uranium	< dl	< 0.2			

CREATININE

	RESULT mg/dL	REFERENCE RANGE	2SD LOW	1SD LOW	MEAN	1SD HIGH	2SD HIGH
Creatinine	30	40- 142					

SPECIMEN DATA

Comments:
Date Collected: 11/3/2003
Date Received: 11/4/2003
Date Completed: 11/10/2003

Method: ICP-MS
<dl: less than detection limit
Provoking Agent:

Collection Period: Random
Volume:
Provocation: POST PROVOCATIVE

URINE TOXIC METALS

DOCTOR'S DATA INC

LAB#:
PATIENT:
SEX: Male
AGE: 6

CLIENT#: 27080
DOCTOR: Amy Yasko, ND
Holistic Health
Po Box 309
Bethel, ME 04217

POTENTIALLY TOXIC METALS

METALS	RESULT µg/g CREAT	REFERENCE RANGE	WITHIN REFERENCE RANGE	ELEVATED	VERY ELEVATED
Aluminum	< dl	< 60			
Antimony	< dl	< 1.5			
Arsenic	38	< 130			
Beryllium	< dl	< 0.6			
Bismuth	< dl	< 20			
Cadmium	< dl	< 2			
Lead	< dl	< 18			
Mercury	10	< 5			
Nickel	< dl	< 15			
Platinum	< dl	< 1			
Thallium	0.7	< 1.1			
Thorium	< dl	< 0.5			
Tin	< dl	< 15			
Tungsten	< dl	< 1.5			
Uranium	< dl	< 0.2			

CREATININE

	RESULT mg/dL	REFERENCE RANGE	2SD LOW	1SD LOW	MEAN	1SD HIGH	2SD HIGH
Creatinine	14	40- 142					

SPECIMEN DATA

Comments:

Date Collected:	3/23/2004	Method:	ICP-MS	Collection Period:	Random
Date Received:	3/31/2004	<dl:	less than detection limit	Volume:	
Date Completed:	4/1/2004	Provoking Agent:		Provocation:	

URINE TOXIC METALS

DOCTOR'S DATA INC

LAB#:
PATIENT:
SEX: Male
AGE: 4

CLIENT#: 27080
DOCTOR: Amy Yasko, ND
Holistic Health
Po Box 309
Bethel, ME 04217

POTENTIALLY TOXIC METALS

METALS	RESULT µg/g CREAT	REFERENCE RANGE	WITHIN REFERENCE RANGE	ELEVATED	VERY ELEVATED
Aluminum	< dl	< 35			
Antimony	< dl	< 5			
Arsenic	58	< 100			
Beryllium	< dl	< 0.5			
Bismuth	0.4	< 30			
Cadmium	0.4	< 2			
Lead	< dl	< 15			
Mercury	6.8	< 3			
Nickel	< dl	< 12			
Platinum	< dl	< 2			
Thallium	0.3	< 14			
Thorium	0.1	< 12			
Tin	1.4	< 6			
Tungsten	0.4	< 23			
Uranium	0.1	< 1			

CREATININE

	RESULT mg/dL	REFERENCE RANGE	2SD LOW	1SD LOW	MEAN	1SD HIGH	2SD HIGH
Creatinine	23	21- 76					

SPECIMEN DATA

Comments:
Date Collected: 9/20/2003
Date Received: 9/22/2003
Date Completed: 9/24/2003

Method: ICP-MS
<dl: less than detection limit
Provoking Agent:

Collection Period: Random
Volume:
Provocation:

FECAL METALS

DOCTOR'S DATA INC

LAB#:
PATIENT:
SEX: Male
AGE: 8

CLIENT#: 27080
DOCTOR: Amy Yasko, ND
Holistic Health
Po Box 309
Bethel, ME 04217

POTENTIALLY TOXIC METALS

METALS	RESULT mg/kg	REFERENCE RANGE	PERCENTILE 68th 95th
Mercury	< dl	<.05 w/o amalgams*	
Mercury	< dl	< .5 with amalgams*	
Antimony	0.042	< 0.080	
Arsenic	1.00	< 0.30	
Beryllium	0.011	< 0.009	
Bismuth	0.008	< 0.050	
Cadmium	0.11	< 0.50	
Copper	24	< 60	
Lead	0.17	< 0.50	
Nickel	3.4	< 8.0	
Platinum	< dl	< 0.003	
Thallium	0.011	< 0.020	
Tungsten	0.120	< 0.090	
Uranium	0.146	< 0.120	

% WATER CONTENT

	RESULT % H_2O	EXPECTED RANGE	2SD LOW 1SD LOW MEAN 72.5% 1SD HIGH 2SD HIGH
% WATER CONTENT	64	60-85%	

FECAL METALS

DOCTOR'S DATA INC

LAB#:
PATIENT:
SEX: Male
AGE: 8

CLIENT#: 27080
DOCTOR: Amy Yasko, ND
Holistic Health
Po Box 309
Bethel, ME 04217

POTENTIALLY TOXIC METALS

METALS	RESULT mg/kg	REFERENCE RANGE	PERCENTILE 68th 95th
Mercury	0.158	<.05 w/o amalgams*	
Mercury	0.158	< .5 with amalgams*	
Antimony	0.026	< 0.080	
Arsenic	0.09	< 0.30	
Beryllium	< dl	< 0.009	
Bismuth	0.008	< 0.050	
Cadmium	0.02	< 0.50	
Copper	8	< 60	
Lead	0.17	< 0.50	
Nickel	0.7	< 8.0	
Platinum	0.003	< 0.003	
Thallium	< dl	< 0.020	
Tungsten	0.018	< 0.090	
Uranium	0.088	< 0.120	

% WATER CONTENT

	RESULT % H_2O	EXPECTED RANGE	2SD LOW 1SD LOW MEAN 72.5% 1SD HIGH 2SD HIGH
% WATER CONTENT	98.2	60-85%	

FECAL METALS

DOCTOR'S DATA INC

LAB#:
PATIENT:
SEX: Male
AGE: 4

CLIENT#: 27080
DOCTOR: Amy Yasko, ND
Holistic Health
Po Box 309
Bethel, ME 04217

POTENTIALLY TOXIC METALS

METALS	RESULT mg/kg	REFERENCE RANGE	PERCENTILE 68th 95th
Mercury	0.008	<.05 w/o amalgams*	
Mercury	0.008	< .5 with amalgams*	
Antimony	0.126	< 0.08	
Arsenic	0.12	< 0.3	
Beryllium	< dl	< 0.009	
Bismuth	0.036	< 0.05	
Cadmium	0.95	< 0.5	
Copper	40	< 60	
Lead	0.19	< 0.5	
Nickel	4.8	< 8.00	
Platinum	< dl	< 0.003	
Thallium	0.023	< 0.02	
Tungsten	0.022	< 0.09	
Uranium	0.064	< 0.12	

% WATER CONTENT

	RESULT % H_2O	EXPECTED RANGE	2SD LOW 1SD LOW MEAN 72.5% 1SD HIGH 2SD HIGH
% WATER CONTENT	79.4	60-85%	

FECAL METALS

DOCTOR'S DATA INC

LAB#:
PATIENT:
SEX: Male
AGE: 4

CLIENT#: 27080
DOCTOR: Amy Yasko, ND
Holistic Health
Po Box 309
Bethel, ME 04217

POTENTIALLY TOXIC METALS

METALS	RESULT mg/kg	REFERENCE RANGE	PERCENTILE 68th 95th
Mercury	0.019	<.05 w/o amalgams*	
Mercury	0.019	< .5 with amalgams*	
Antimony	0.093	< 0.08	
Arsenic	0.30	< 0.3	
Beryllium	0.026	< 0.009	
Bismuth	0.052	< 0.05	
Cadmium	0.79	< 0.5	
Copper	120	< 60	
Lead	0.54	< 0.5	
Nickel	8.4	< 8.00	
Platinum	< dl	< 0.003	
Thallium	0.031	< 0.02	
Tungsten	0.044	< 0.09	
Uranium	0.112	< 0.12	

% WATER CONTENT

	RESULT % H_2O	EXPECTED RANGE	2SD LOW 1SD LOW MEAN 72.5% 1SD HIGH 2SD HIGH
% WATER CONTENT	80	60-85%	

FECAL METALS

DOCTOR'S DATA INC.

LAB#
PATIENT:
SEX: Male
AGE: 4

CLIENT#: 27080
DOCTOR: Amy Yasko, ND
Holistic Health
Po Box 309
Bethel, ME 04217

POTENTIALLY TOXIC METALS

METALS	RESULT mg/kg	REFERENCE RANGE	PERCENTILE 68th 95th
Mercury	0.011	<.05 w/o amalgams*	
Mercury	0.011	< .5 with amalgams*	
Antimony	0.143	< 0.08	
Arsenic	0.25	< 0.3	
Beryllium	0.005	< 0.009	
Bismuth	0.086	< 0.05	
Cadmium	0.57	< 0.5	
Copper	24	< 60	
Lead	0.15	< 0.5	
Nickel	2.1	< 8.00	
Platinum	< dl	< 0.003	
Thallium	0.032	< 0.02	
Tungsten	0.015	< 0.09	
Uranium	0.051	< 0.12	

% WATER CONTENT

	RESULT % H_2O	EXPECTED RANGE	2SD LOW 1SD LOW MEAN 72.5% 1SD HIGH 2SD HIGH
% WATER CONTENT	84.7	60-85%	

Appendix

Supplements & Descriptions

Note: References supporting the use of these supplements can be found at www.holistichealth.com.

Vitamin A- (beta carotene) This vitamin has a bit of a mixed "pedigree". Vitamin A is a fat-soluble vitamin, so it has the potential to accumulate in tissues and cause liver toxicity. Conversely, if an individual has difficulties with fat absorption, they may actually be deficient in Vitamin A. Alcohol can enhance the toxicity of Vitamin A. Elevated levels of Vitamin A are associated with an increased risk of hip fracture in women. On the other hand, Vitamin A is an antioxidant, neutralizing free radicals. There have been some studies, which suggest that high levels of Vitamin A may increase the risk of certain cancers, including breast cancer and lung cancer. However, other studies have shown Vitamin A to be useful in combating cervical cancer. This condition has been correlated with infection by the human papilloma virus. Vitamin A is often recommended for children with autism. This may stem from work in Africa, which found that high doses of Vitamin A were useful in reducing the severity of measles viral infection. Subsequent work has shown that while Vitamin A is useful to help eradicate virus if there is a Vitamin A deficiency, it can actually promote viral transmission if there is no deficiency. This may explain some of the divergent results with the use of Vitamin A. Caution should be used when considering the use of high doses of Vitamin A.

Acidophilus- This is a probiotic, or the natural bacteria that line your intestinal tract. It is important to repopulate your body with normal flora. Acidophilus is one of several types of probiotics. The most basic is simply acidophilus. **Allerdophilus** works in a similar fashion, but is designed for allergic individuals. **Kyodophilus** is a chewable form that works well for young children. **Supremadophilus** is an excellent probiotic. It contains normal flora, FOS, which is basically food to help producing healthy bacteria levels for the normal bacteria grow.

Adrenal Support- Adrenal insufficiency occurs when the adrenals are unable to produce normal amounts of hormones, or when the body has a reduced capacity to deal with chronic stress. A professional health care practitioner who may advise the use of an Adrenal Supplement best diagnoses this condition.

Alpha Lipoic Acid- This helps to increase glutathione in the liver. It supplies a sulfur group to the body. It is also one of the few antioxidants that are able to work in both the water and the fat phases in the body. As a result it is able to help with oxidized cholesterol. It is often used in conjunction with other sulfur containing supplements for heavy metal detoxification when used as part of the diet to maintain healthy blood.

Artichoke- This works well in conjunction with **Yellow Dock** to relieve occasional constipation. It is a nice addition to a daily supplement regime, with or without the yellow dock. It will also help to maintain cholesterol levels that are already in the normal range.

ATP- This can be used as an alternative, or in conjunction with **NADH,** as a source of energy to help with detoxification. Your brain needs adequate stores of ATP in order to detoxify harmful substances.

B Complex- This will help build nerves and form acetylcholine; it should also be used in conjunction with **SAMe** supplementation. B vitamins are particularly critical for memory. They also help to make acetylcholine that has been shown to be correlated with memory issues. B vitamins help the liver, help the body to deal with stress. Stress depletes B vitamins. They are water-soluble; any excess is excreted so B's need to be supplemented on a daily basis. Excess

B's may turn urine a bright yellow- this is fine! It is important to take B vitamins as a complex, as it has been shown that taking a single B vitamin will deplete the levels of the other B vitamin's and this occurs in a dose dependent fashion. For example, a central inflammatory mediator in other neurological inflammation is homocysteine. Lack of particular B's will increase the homocysteine levels in the blood. A general B supplement should help to lower homocysteine levels.

B12- (methylcobolamine) This is one of the B vitamins. Unlike the other B vitamins this form of B is degraded in the stomach so most of it is destroyed when it is swallowed. The individual B12s melt in the mouth like a mint, so they can be absorbed without being degraded. They help to balance glutamate and GABA, and serve as methyl donors. They are great for energy and to fight fatigue. They have been found to help with motion sickness and to calm nervousness. There are reports to suggest that B12 helps to regenerate nerves. It is a good idea to supplement with a variety of forms of B12 simultaneously, using the cyano form, the methyl form, and the hydroxy forms of B12.

Bacopa- This ayurvedic herb works nicely in conjunction with **Gotu Kola**. It has been reported to help with communication between the left and right sides of the brain. Using bacopa with gotu kola has been helpful in terms of communication.

Black cohosh- This herb is useful to offset mild symptoms of menopause. It works well in conjunction with **Vitex** and **Dong Quai**. If that combination is not successful then the product listed as **Natural Estrogen** will often help to remedy symptoms of menopause. It is a good idea to also supplement with **Indole 3 Carbinol** when using black cohosh.

Borage Oil- This is an excellent source of both omega 3 and omega 6 essential fatty acids. Borage Oil works especially well to soothe dry irritated skin. Borage Oil can be taken orally as well as a topical lotion (**Shikai**). Some individuals prefer borage oil to evening primrose oil for "PMS type symptoms" or breast soreness associated with menstrual cycles, and found that it is more effective for these conditions.

Boswellia- It supports joint health and maintenance. It works best as part of a "trio" along with **Curcumin** and **Nettle**.

Branched Chain Amino Acids- This helps to protect the blood brain barrier, and to control glutamate. This supplement should not be used if a maple syrup smell is apparent in the urine.

Broccoli- Most of us do not eat enough broccoli, so it is nice to be able to enhance our levels with a supplement. Broccoli is a wonderful source of sulfur. The more sulfur the better, especially when it comes to neurological health.

Buffer pH- This supplement is best used in combination with a pH kit. This way you can determine the pH of your urine or saliva before attempting to balance your pH. This supplement when used in conjunction with a pH kit will aid in maintaining proper PH balance in the body.

Burdock Root- This is an especially good supplement to purify and detoxify the body in a gentle fashion. We are all exposed to so many stressors and toxins in our everyday lives. This is an easy way to try to undo some of that damage on a daily basis.

Burpleurum- This has been reported to be helpful in supporting the liver.

Vitamin C- This helps with the absorption of nutrients in the brain, thus increasing their ability to cross the blood brain barrier. Vitamin C also helps to regenerate glutathione, a critical detoxification substance that is made by the liver. The more Vitamin C, the better, as long as it doesn't cause problems with loose bowels.

Calcium- The best calcium supplements contain calcium, magnesium, Vitamin D and Vitamin K. A number of practitioners are not huge supporters of the current trend toward massive doses of calcium. Based on expertise with neurological inflammation, large doses of calcium can actually be detrimental to the body. All the calcium in the world will not get to where it is needed in the body without sufficient Vitamin D and Vitamin K. Many people who believe they are calcium deficient are actually low in the fat-soluble Vitamins D and K. As we age, our ability to break down fats and assimilate these vitamins may decrease. Taking high doses of calcium can also deplete the body's stores of magnesium. Magnesium is helpful for the heart, for blood sugar levels and for muscle cramping. Calcium supplements are available that contain Vitamin D and Vitamin K to help with the absorption of calcium, as well as a ratio of 750 mg of calcium to 500 mg of magnesium to help keep these mineral in balance. For those who desire a 1:1 ratio of calcium to magnesium, you can add additional 250mg magnesium. While there have been reports that calcium helps with weight loss, it has also been reported in the literature that there is an inverse relationship between osteoporosis and hormone sensitive cancers. What this study implies is that the higher the bone density, the greater the risk of beast cancer. This is another reason to use moderation with respect to calcium.

Candex- There have been reports of great success with the use of this supplement to help balance flora. It should be used in conjunction with a number of other supplements designed to restore a balance to the normal flora in the body.

Carnitine- This has been found to be helpful for the heart and for the liver. It also is useful in converting fat into energy, increasing the energy in the mitochondria that are the energy storage centers in your cells, and helping to maintain cholesterol levels that are already in the normal range.

Carnosine + Rosemary- Carnosine has been reported to help break down beta amyloid plaque and to limit the hexamer reaction in the body. It may also help to reduce both iron and copper in the system, thereby aiding in the balance of the copper/zinc ratio. Rosemary helps to keep the Carnosine intact so that it can do its job. Taken together, this combination works really well.

Cascara sagrada- This supplement is excellent for those with sluggish bowels. Cascara is reported to be non-habit forming, so it can be useful for those who are trying to break a laxative dependency. It has also been described to strengthen the colon and help promote and maintain its health. This supplement works well in conjunction with **Artichoke** and **Yellow Dock**.

Cell Food- A few drops of this liquid supplement can be added to a drink or a glass of water to provide a wide range of minerals, enzymes and other nutrients. Cell Food is a nice accompaniment to a detoxification program or a chelation program to ensure that you do not become depleted in minerals.

Chamomile- This is traditionally used as a calming herb and for help with sleep. It is actually a natural source of calcium. However, chamomile also helps to maintain healthy levels of the enzyme control MAPkinase. This is a good supplement for those who are concerned about their calcium intake, yet at the same time would like to prevent inflammation as a result of calcium.

Cherry Extract- This is an excellent supplement when fresh tart cherries are out of season. This supplement is exceedingly helpful for high uric acid conditions.

Choachol- This is a gall bladder supplement that has a simple yet effective suggested use. It has been reported to help individuals who have had their gall bladders removed. A number of individuals have had tremendous success using this supplement to counter the "dumping syndrome" often encountered after gall bladder removal.

Choline- This is a specific supplement that is in the B family. Choline will work to directly help to synthesize additional acetylcholine. While there is choline in the B complex, additional choline is a good idea in individuals with memory problems associated with aging.

Chondroitin- Many people like to take a combination of glucosamine plus chondroitin for joint support. Others prefer a separate chondroitin supplement that is formulated to be well absorbed. Many chondroitin supplements or combination supplements are of a high molecular weight and are not easily absorbed. It is important to use low molecular weight chondroitin. It also works well with **Glucosamine/MSM** supplements.

Citrimax- This contains **Chromium Picolinate** to help with blood sugar, as well as garcinia, which is an extract from citrus fruit. It has been reported to help stimulate the metabolism and aid in weight management. This supplement works well taken in conjunction with a **Green Tea** oral supplement.

Cod Liver Oil- This is an excellent supplement for those who want to support the liver, or those who have issues with occasional constipation. Many individuals prefer a gel cap supplement, which can be swallowed, over liquid forms of cod liver oil.

Collagen- This supplement is often utilized for skin health, as well as to support joint health. It is often helpful for individuals who need joint support when a **glucosamine/chondroitin** supplement has been unable to make a difference.

Collinsonia- (otherwise known as **Stone root)** This herb is helpful for strengthening the veins. Many individuals prefer this supplement to butchers broom for this purpose, as it should not create potential blood pressure issues as can occur with butcher's broom. Horse chestnut is another good supplement for vein strength. Horse chestnut is also available as a topical cream. It can be used in conjunction with collinsonia. For those with blood pressure issues the safest approach would be an oral collinsonia supplement with or without topical cream.

Complete Vitamin and Ultra Antioxidant- This includes vitamins, antioxidants, and minerals to lay the nutritional groundwork. It is preferable to use a complete vitamin that is specially formulated with neurological inflammation in mind. It should have no copper, no iron and limited calcium relative to magnesium. In addition to all the essential vitamins and minerals it should contain milk thistle, N-acetyl cysteine, and selenium to help the body make glutathione (a critical antioxidant made in the liver). It should also include pine bark extract (pycnogenol) to protect the glutamate receptors, and taurine to help balance glutamate and GABA.

Colostrum- This helps to support the immune system. Colostrum is particularly helpful for stomach and intestinal health.

CoQ10- This can be thought of as the "currency" that the cells of your body trade in rather than money. As a result, it is important for your cells to have adequate stores of CoQ10. This will help with energy, build new nerves and help with membrane fluidity. Based on a recent NIH study, more is better with CoQ10. CoQ10 is an important antioxidant for oxidative damage in the body, including in the fat phase, not simply the water phase in the cells. There have been reports that indicate that low levels of CoQ10 are a factor in congestive heart failure. Any individual taking statin drugs should be supplementing with CoQ10 on a daily basis.

Cox 2 Support Mixture- This is a combination of a number of supplements that are reported to help support fluid balance in joints. Natural joint support supplements include phellodendron, tumeric ginger, white willow, boswellia, devil's claw, green tea, bromelain, papain, protease, grape seed, rosemary, quercetin and polygonum.

Cranberry- This supplement has a reputation for being helpful for urinary tract health. There is literature to support its ability to maintain flora balance. Cranberry works well in conjunction with a number of other supplements that may have antimicrobial properties. One group that works extremely well together is **Oregon grape, Neem, Myrrh, Golden Seal, Cranberry, and Oregamax, +/- Uva Ursi.**

Curbita- This is an extract from pumpkin. There are reports to suggest that pumpkin extract helps to strengthen the bladder muscles.

Curcumin- This is a truly excellent supplement. It is a natural promoter of joint/cartilage health, which is helpful to those looking for joint support. It also works nicely as part of a "trio" along with **Boswellia** and **Nettle**. Curcumin has also been reported to be helpful in promoting colon and skin health. It serves as a methyl donor.

Vitamin D- This can be taken in winter or in cloudy regions to supplement the Vitamin D in the General Vitamin. Adequate levels of Vitamin D are important to immune health. A correlation has been found between areas of the country with reduced sun exposure and healthy levels of Vitamin D.

Dandelion Leaf- This supplement taken several times daily is very helpful to support the kidneys and bladder. It works nicely in combination with taurine and SAMe with a B complex for kidney health.

Dandelion Root- While dandelion leaf is lovely for the kidneys, dandelion root helps to support the liver. The liver is one of the most important organs in the body. It is responsible for detoxification in the body, and the liver synthesizes glutathione, which is critical for detoxification and immune support. Supporting the liver is therefore of utmost importance. Dandelion root works well with **Milk Thistle** for liver support.

DHEA- For years this supplement was touted as the fountain of youth, helping to offset aging. It is true that as we age, our DHEA levels decline along with estrogen or testosterone. It has also been reported to be helpful in a variety of immune boosting mechanisms. DHEA can be of use when an individual has low levels of DHEA. However, it is not wise to supplement with DHEA unless you have confirmed the fact that your levels are low and in need of supplementation. Taking a supplement that can increase hormone levels is a double-edged sword. If you need it then it may be extremely helpful to supplement. If you do not need it, you may run the risk of increasing hormone levels to a point where you could cause abnormal growth in your body.

Digestive Enzymes- There are two types of digestive enzymes that work especially well when used together, **Super Digestive Enzymes** and **Ultra Dairy**. This pair of enzymes help with bloating, the digestion of fats, support the pancreas, help with minor blood sugar issues, and may help with acid neutralization. It is a good idea to take one of each with every meal.

DMG (dimethyl glycine)- The glycine can stimulate the glutamate activity when glutamate is still in excess. As the glutamate is more under control, then the DMG will work well in conjunction with GABA. DMG is also a very good methyl donor. Methylation is important for autism. DMG can also be helpful for neurological health.

Dong Quai- This supplement is useful to offset symptoms of menopause. It works well in conjunction with vitex and black cohosh. If that combination is not successful then the product listed as Natural Estrogen will often help. As with black cohosh, this supplement may be useful in stimulating language. It is best used in conjunction with indole 3 carbinol.

Dopa 400- This natural source of dopa is derived from Mucuna pruriens, or the Velvet Bean. This supplement is helpful for individuals who want to supplement their natural dopamine levels. Imbalances in dopamine levels are known to be a problem in Parkinson's disease. Dopamine imbalances have also been implicated in autism, addictive behaviors and in ADD.

Vitamin E- This is a well-known supplement taken as an antioxidant to help with heart health, prostate health, and perhaps most importantly to regenerate glutathione. Vitamin E is part of a family of supplements known as tocopherols. Vitamin E that is a combination of mixed tocopherols has been reported to be more effective than individual Vitamin E supplements.

Echinacea- This is a classic herb that is used to support the immune system. It is most effective if used as a trio, in conjunction with **Elderberry** and **Goldenseal**. Echinacea should not be used as a daily supplement. Rather, it should only be used when needed. Individuals with allergies should be cautious in their use of this herb; individuals with autoimmune conditions should avoid the use of Echinacea.

EDTA- This supplement works extremely well in chelating metals without the side effects seen with other chelating agents. There is also extensive literature available concerning the use of EDTA to help support the heart.

EFA (essential fatty acids) + Neuromins- This combination provides a ideal ratio of omega 3/6/9.

Elderberry- This herb is excellent for supporting the gut.

Fenugreek- This supplement will help heal the gut, increase milk production for breast-feeding and help balance sugar levels when used as part of the diet.

Feverfew- This herb helps in the prevention of migraine headaches.

Fish Oil- Fish oil is helpful for maintaining cholesterol levels that are already in the normal range.

Folic Acid- While folic acid is generally included in most B complexes, it is worth considering additional supplementation of this particular B vitamin. Folic acid helps to reduce homocysteine. High levels of homocysteine do not promote heart health. Folic acid is important in helping to prevent neural tube defects. It is also involved in the important methylation pathways in the body. In some cases, alternative sources of folic acid are necessary due to blocks in the pathway of folate metabolism. In these cases the use of **FolaPro (5 methyl folate)**, and or **Folinic Acid** should be considered.

GABA- This is a calming neurotransmitter in the body that helps to balance glutamate. It should be useful to help decrease stress, and increase speech, eye contact, and social interactions. GABA comes in several forms and it will be a bit of trial and error to determine which is best. **GABA Calm** seems to work well for many individuals during the day; it melts in the mouth like a lozenge. For those who do not like the taste or prefer to swallow a pill, **GABA** is also available as a supplement to be swallowed. **ZEN** (GABA and Theanine) is nice to take later in the evening as it helps with sleep and stress.

Garlic- This has the potential to do many wonderful things: help control cholesterol, help the liver, maintain cholesterol levels that are already in the normal range and participate in sulfur reactions in body.

Ginkgo- This has been reported to increase blood flow to the brain and to protect from damage due to nitric oxide. It may also help to slow the breakdown of dopamine as it has been reported to act as an MAO-B inhibitor. Ginkgo should be used with caution in individuals with blood pressure issues.

Glucosamine/MSM- Many people like to take a combination of **glucosamine/chondroitin** for joint support. Others prefer a separate **chondroitin** supplement that is formulated to be well absorbed. Many **chondroitin** supplements or combination supplements are of a high molecular weight and are not easily absorbed.

Glucose support- There are a number of nutritional supplements and herbs that can be used as part of the diet to help maintain healthy blood sugar levels. Combinations are available that include many of the herbs that may help, such as Vitamin E, magnesium, zinc, manganese, chromium, lagerstroemia speciosa, bitter melon, gymnema sylvestre, vanadyl sulfate, Jerusalem artichoke, fenugreek, milk thistle, ginkgo biloba, bilberry, alpha lipoic acid, citric bioflavonoids.

Glutathione- This is one of the most important supplements made by the body. It is helpful in programs designed to promote immune and neurological health. There are also reports that suggest that glutathione is useful for cystic fibrosis. If glutathione is not specially formulated it degrades in the stomach if it is swallowed.

Goldenseal- This works well in conjunction with a number of other supplements that may have antimicrobial properties. One group that works extremely well together is **Oregon Grape, Neem, Myrrh, Goldenseal, Cranberry, and Oregamax, +/- Uva Ursi.**

Gotu Kola- This ayurvedic herb is excellent in conjunction with **Bacopa**. It has been reported to help with communication between the left and right sides of the brain. Using bacopa with gotu kola has been helpful with communication.

Grape Seed Extract- This is reported to help to control glutamate by protecting the glutamate receptors and to support nerve health in the brain. It works well in conjunction with pycnogenol.

Green Tea- There are so many good things about green tea as a supplement. It has been described as helpful in everything from immune health, skin health, to increasing the metabolism for weight management.

Guarana- This nutritional supplement has many times the level of caffeine found in coffee. Caffeine is not always a negative. It may be helpful for many individuals who need extra pick-up. There is also information to suggest that caffeine can help with apoptosis.

Guggulipid-Ayur- This is useful in supporting the thyroid, for adolescent non-cystic acne, and to support the immune system.

Gymnema-Ayur- This is an ayurvedic herb that helps to support the pancreas health, and can be used as part of the diet to help maintain blood sugar levels. If used on a regular basis this works well for children who become "hyper" after ingesting sugar.

Hawthorn- This supplement is often thought of as a general heart tonic for overall heart wellness. It is a good idea to supplement with this herb for optimal heart health. This supplement works nicely in combination with **CoQ10.**

Helix- This nutrient provides breast health support.

Hops- There is literature that supports the use of hops to help balance hormone levels. It has been reported to help to convert testosterone to estrogen. This may be helpful in hormonal imbalances and in adolescent non-cystic acne. It would be wise to take **Indole 3 Carbinol** and or **Broccoli** in conjunction with hops to help keep the estrogen of the healthier type.

Horse chestnut- This is often used to support weak veins. It works nicely when used in conjunction with **Collinsonia**.

Horsetail grass- This is reportedly a rich source of silica. Horsetail grass can be helpful in aiding in bone health development. It may also be useful in helping to detoxify aluminum from the body.

Indole 3 Carbinol- This supplement has been described to help keep estrogen as the "healthy" type in the body. This can be taken as a daily supplement and is helpful for breast health.

Inositol and IP6- Inositol has been reported to be useful for helping to control obsessive behaviors. Inositol is also useful for supplementation to the muscles. Some practitioners prefer IP6 to standard inositol.

Juniper Berry- This has been described as being useful for urinary tract health. It is a reasonably strong supplement so it is not generally suggested for everyday use. A potentially more important use of Juniper Berry may be in breast health.

Vitamin K- Since glycosylation occurs as a result of sugar hooking onto protein in an incorrect fashion, supplements that help with sugar regulation should also help to decrease glycosylation. Vitamin K helps to control sugar. It also helps with bleeding and bruising. Vitamin K is a fat-soluble vitamin but it is not stored in the body like the other fat-soluble vitamins. Vitamin K needs to be made by the body or taken as a supplement on a daily, or every other day, basis. Some studies show that Vitamin K is more powerful than Vitamin E and coenzyme Q10 for scavenging free radicals and in other studies Vitamin K by itself completely protected the liver from free radicals. Vitamin E and glutathione protect Vitamin K's antioxidant effect.

Kelp- This is a rich source of iodine. Many years ago the purpose behind putting iodine in salt was precisely to help prevent iodine deficiency. In today's society, where many of us restrict our salt intake, we may be lacking in iodine. Kelp can be used as another means of replacing iodine rather than table salt. Sufficient iodine is important for the proper functioning of the thyroid gland.

Lactoferrin- This is an all-natural extract from milk.

Liv-Ora- This whole organ extract support for the liver.

Lobelia- This is a powerful and potentially dangerous supplement. It can be helpful for breaking addictive behaviors including cigarette smoking. The best idea is to use minimal quantities of this supplement, only for as long as is necessary.

Lutein Plus- This supplement is a lovely combination of several supplements that have been reported to be helpful in supporting eye health. It includes lutein, zeaxanithin, bilberry, and a bit of vitamin E.

Lycopene- There are a number of studies to suggest that lycopene is helpful for the prostate and for cancer prevention.

Lysine- This amino acid has been reported to help with viral infections.

Magnesium- This helps to block the flow of calcium into the neurons. Some individuals find that they have loose stools from too much magnesium. Conversely, magnesium is useful for constipation. Magnesium is helpful for the heart, for blood sugar levels, PMS, for muscle cramping and for lung health. There is some concern about the excessive amounts of calcium that many individuals are ingesting. It may be causing magnesium deficiencies, which may be even more dangerous.

Malic acid- The use of malic acid with magnesium is a good idea for individuals in need of immune support. It is also helpful in chelating aluminum.

Marshmallow- This supplement can be used to help soothe inflamed areas. It works well for everything from throat health to urinary tract health. It works best as an addition to other more targeted supplement.

Mastica gum- Mastica gum can be helpful for individuals looking for skin, stomach, gastric and intestinal health support.

Melatonin- This supplement is useful for aiding in sleep. Melatonin is also reported to be a powerful antioxidant in the brain. Several types of melatonin are available - **immediate release** is suggested for those who occasionally have trouble falling asleep. **Time release** is suggested for those who can fall asleep, but wake up during the night and can't get back to sleep. And a combination product, **Natural Sleep** is suggested for those who occasionally have trouble both falling asleep and staying asleep.

Melissa- This herb has been suggested to help relieve cold sores.

Milk Thistle- The liver is a central organ that is involved in contributing to neurological health. There is milk thistle in some general vitamins; however, in this case, more is better. Milk Thistle helps to balance liver enzyme levels, improves glutathione levels, builds new nerves and helps maintain liver health.

Minerals- There are several types of mineral supplementation, **Bio Nativus** liquid trace mineral drops that can be put in drinking water, and an **Ultra Mineral** supplement that can be swallowed.

Mistletoe- There have been reports in the literature that suggests the use of mistletoe may be helpful in immune health. It is best used as part of a more comprehensive program that includes a number of supplements to achieve optimal results.

Moducare- This supplement has been reported to help with viral infections.

Mycoceutics (mushrooms + beta glucan)- There are a number of mushroom supplements on the market. Products that have a wonderful combination of a variety of mushrooms, in addition to beta-glucan, seem to work best. This supplement should be used as part of a more complete program to support the immune system.

Myrrh- This works well in conjunction with a number of other supplements that may have antimicrobial properties. One group that works extremely well together is **Oregon Grape, Neem, Myrrh, Golden Seal, Cranberry, Oregamax +/- Uva Ursi.** Myrrh has also been reported to be helpful for low platelet levels. 1

N-acetyl-cysteine- This helps the liver to make glutathione. NAC is particularly good for the lungs and has been found to be useful for respiratory health and when used as part of the diet to help maintain healthy blood sugar levels. It should always be taken with Vitamin C.

NADH- This is important in energy production, particularly in the Krebs cycle. It is often useful to supplement with NADH if you are using glutathione as it helps to regenerate the glutathione to the reduced form without depleting the body's stores of NADH. This supplement is useful for neurological health.

Natural Estrogen- This supplement will often help to remedy symptoms of menopause. It works well in conjunction with topical **progesterone cream**.

Neem- This works well in conjunction with a number of other supplements that may have antimicrobial properties. One group that works extremely well together is **Oregon Grape, Neem, Myrrh, Goldenseal, and Cranberry, Oregamax +/- Uva Ursi.**

Nettle- This works nicely to help maintain joint fluid balance, promote joint health and skin health. It works best as part of a "trio" along with **curcumin** and **boswellia**. Nettle is also a good source of boron, which is excellent for the bones.

Neuromins- This is a wonderful source of omega 3 fatty acids. It is a good idea to use Neuromins, or DHA in conjunction with a complete EFA for the optimal balance of omega 3, 6, 9 fatty acids.

No-Phenol- This supplement is designed to help individuals who have difficulty ingesting substances that contain phenol molecules.

Ora-Triplex- A whole organ support for the immune system, to include the spleen, liver, and thymus extracts.

Oregamax- This works well in conjunction with a number of other supplements that may have antimicrobial properties. One group that works extremely well together is **Oregon Grape, Neem, Myrrh, Goldenseal, and Cranberry, Oregamax +/- Uva Ursi.**

Oregon Grape- This works well in conjunction with a number of other supplements that may have antimicrobial properties. One group that works extremely well together is **Oregon Grape, Neem, Myrrh, Goldenseal, Cranberry, Oregamax +/- Uva Ursi.**

Oxydrene- According to the available literature this supplement should be useful in increasing oxygenation in the body. In addition to adequate ATP, your brain needs sufficient oxygenation to protect itself and to detoxify harmful substances. Oxydrene has been found to have positive effects on neurological inflammation.

PABA (Para Amino Benzoic Acid)- While this B vitamin is included in general B complexes it is worth considering additional supplementation of PABA in individuals who want additional thyroid support.

Pancreas-Ora- A whole organ extract support for the pancreas.

Pantothenic Acid- While this B vitamin is included in general B complexes it is worth considering additional supplementation of Pantothenic Acid to help maintain cholesterol levels already within the normal range.

Papaya- This is a very tasty chewable supplement that can help with digestion. Papaya is a rich source of enzymes that have been described to be useful for skin as well as for digestion.

Paradex- This is the best combination of supplements that have been found to help control parasites.

Parsley- This herb has been described to have gentle diuretic and laxative properties.

Pau d Arco- This works best as part of a more complete program to support the immune system.

Petadolex- This is an excellent source of butterbur. There are a number of articles describing the use of **butterbur** to help alleviate migraine headaches and severe allergies.

Phaseolamin- This is an extract from the white kidney bean that has been reported to help decrease fat absorption. This is a nice supplement to use in conjunction with an overall weight management program.

Phosphatidyl serine- This increases acetylcholine as well as decreases stress and helps with membrane fluidity that may be compromised due to oxidized cholesterol. This is a membrane component that helps to coat nerves. It functions to protect nerves in a similar fashion to the way the rubber or plastic coating insulates electric wiring. A good source of phosphatidyl serine, phosphatidyl choline and phosphatidyl inositol.

Placenta-Ora- A whole organ extract support that contains placental extracts.

Policosanol- This helps to maintain cholesterol levels that are already in the normal range and to increase membrane fluidity.

Primal Defense- This supplement is a nice accompaniment to a detoxification program or a chelation program to ensure that you do not become depleted in a variety of nutrients and provides a full spectrum of organisms to promote and then maintain an optimal bowel flora. It works far better with appropriate fiber support such as **Beyond Fiber**.

Progesterone Cream- This topical cream can be used to help balance hormone levels.

Psyllium Husk- This is often used by individuals with bowel or constipation issues. Another excellent supplement combination for constipation is artichoke, yellow dock, and +/- cascara sagrada as needed. However, psyllium husk is a traditional standby that will help.

Pycnogenol- This can be used to help to control glutamate by protecting the glutamate receptors, as well as to help revitalize nerves. Pycnogenol is also reported to help strengthen veins.

Quercetin- This may help to prevent histamine release. Quercetin helps to retain the levels of carnosine in the body. Quercetin can also be useful for promoting eye health. Quercetin is also reported to help lower uric acid levels, and be helpful for prostate health.

Relaxation- This supplement is a combination of a number of calming and relaxing herbs to help with stress reduction or tension, which includes Theanine, oat, magnolia, chamomile, lemon balm, valerian, scullcap, hops, passionflower, magnesium, and B-6. This combination may help to increase the number of GABA receptors.

Rosemary- This herb is reported to be helpful for memory, and to help increase glutathione levels. Rosemary also helps to keep the **Carnosine** intact so that it can function properly. This combination works really well when taken together.

Rhubarb- This herb is reported to be useful in helping to stem bleeding problems. There is also literature that supports its use to help aid in occasional constipation without causing diarrhea.

SAMe (s-adenosyl methionine)- This is wonderful for the liver. SAMe is also a methyl donor and a sulfur donor for the following reactions in the body. The sulfur donating function is important for detoxification. SAMe is also useful to help the body get rid of excess ammonia. Because SAMe can increase serotonin levels, it can help to elevate the mood. High doses of SAMe are also reported to be highly effective for joint support. A complete B complex should be taken with each SAMe.

Saw Palmetto- This supplement should be considered as a part of a daily health regime for males.

Saw Palmetto Plus Pygeum- This supplement is similar to the standard saw palmetto with a few additional ingredients that may benefit older men.

Selenium- This is an important mineral helping to recycle the glutathione in your body. Selenium can be toxic in high doses, so this is not a case of more is better.

Serraflazyme- This supplement is reported to help break down excess mucous. It can be particularly helpful for those who suffer from chronic mucous build up, or during the winter months when congestion can be an issue.

SerenAid- This is often used as a digestive aid for individuals on a GFCF diet, those unable to digest gluten and casein. SerenAid is also another name for DPP-IV, which is a soluble peptidase involved in immune regulation. This enzyme may also be helpful in supporting the immune system. There is a report in the literature that DDP-IV may be helpful in melanoma.

Slippery Elm- This supplement works well for irritated areas.

Soy Isoflavone- There has been a great deal of literature to support the use of soy supplements. Supplementation with soy is best used in moderation.

Spirulina- The use of this blue/green algae works nicely in conjunction with MGN3 or IP6. There are articles to suggest that Spirulina helps to move natural killer cells from the blood stream into the tissues. Combining supplements that are described to help increase natural killer cell activity, with a supplement to move these immune surveillance cells into the tissues, would be using these supplements to their best advantage.

St. Johns Wort- This supplement is a classic in terms of its use for mood, stress and other emotional issues. Other supplements that may work better for emotional conditions are **SAMe** with a **B complex** or one of the **GABA** supplements.

Taurine- This is an amino acid that is not considered as an essential amino acid in the body. However, individuals who do not eat a lot of red meat are deficient in taurine. Taurine may be useful to the liver by increasing bile output. This helps in the digestion and assimilation of fats and fat-soluble vitamins. Taurine is very useful in controlling imbalances in glutamate and GABA. It may be that taurine is helpful in curtailing the rapid outpouring of taurine is reported to be useful in promoting kidney health maintaining blood pressure levels that are already with in the normal range and when used as part of the diet to maintain healthy blood sugar levels.

Theanine- This is the calming component from green tea. It mimics glutamate and can help protect against excessive glutamate levels.

Thyroid/L-tyrosine- This supplement helps to support the thyroid. This particular combination supplement seems to work better than plain l-tyrosine supplements.

Tonalin (Conjugated Linoleic Acid)- This supplement is often used in conjunction with a weight management program. CLA has been reported to help the body to burn fat.

Transfer Factor- This supplement is excellent for helping to support the immune system.

Trehalose- This is a natural sugar that has been found to decrease the formation of glutamate aggregates.

Uva Ursi- This works well in conjunction with a number of other supplements that may help healthy microbial support. One group that works extremely well together is **Oregon Grape, Neem, Myrrh, Golden Seal, Cranberry, and Oregamax, +/- Uva Ursi.** It is best to use Uva Ursi for two to three weeks and then discontinue it for two to three weeks.

Vinpocetine- This helps to increase circulation to the brain and to remove excess calcium from the brain. It can also act to inhibit microtubule formation and may therefore be useful in triggering apoptosis or programmed cell death (a natural pruning process in cells to eliminate damaged cells).

Vital Yew- This product is available as a supplement, which can be taken orally, and as a topical cream.

Vitex- This helps to balance the levels of estrogen and progesterone. Vitex is useful to offset symptoms of menopause, as well as to offset symptoms of PMS. For symptoms of menopause it works well in conjunction with black cohosh and dong quai. If that combination is not successful then the product listed as **Natural Estrogen** will often help to remedy more severe symptoms.

Yellow Dock- An excellent combination to relieve constipation is **Artichoke** in conjunction with **Yellow Dock**. **Yellow Dock** is a nice addition to a daily supplement regime, with or without the **Artichoke**.

Zinc- This helps to block the flow of calcium into the neurons. Zinc works well for people who cannot tolerate magnesium. However, zinc is a double-edged sword; too much zinc will cause glutamate release. It is best to keep zinc at 25-40 mg per day.

Sources of Excitotoxins

monosodium glutamate
nutrasweet/aspartame
malted barely flour
glutamate
hydrolyzed protein
malt extract
natural flavor(s)
hydrolyzed vegetable protein
malt flavoring(s)
natural flavoring(s)
hydrolyzed plant protein
malted barley/barley malt
maltodextrin
hydrolyzed oat flour
malted anything
carrageenan
hydrolyze anything
textured protein
gelatin
sodium caseinate
guar gum
spice(s)
smoke flavoring(s)
calcium caseinate
whey protein concentrate
plant protein extract l-cysteine
chicken/pork/beef “flavoring” whey protein
chicken/pork/beef “base” whey protein isolate

seasoning(s)
caseinate
soy protein
seasoned salt
disodium guanylate
soy protein concentrate
dough conditioner(s)
disodium inosinate
soy protein isolate
yeast extract
disodium caseinate
soy extract
soy sauce
autolyzed yeast
autolyzed yeast extract
autolyzed anything
bouillon
broth
stock
soup base
vegetable gum
kombu extract
ajinomoto

Sources of MSG

Definite Sources of MSG

- Hydrolyzed Protein or Hydrolyzed Oat Flour
- Sodium Caseinate or Calcium Caseinate
- Autolyzed Yeast or Yeast Extract
- Gelatin
- Glutamic Acid
- Monosodium Glutamate

Possible Sources of MSG

- Textured Protein
- Carrageenan or Vegetable Gum
- Seasonings or Spices
- Flavorings or Natural Flavorings
- Chicken, Beef, Pork, Smoke Flavorings
- Bouillon, Broth or Stock
- Barley Malt, Malt Extract, Malt Flavoring
- Whey Protein, Whey Protein Isolate or Concentrate
- Soy Protein, Soy Protein Isolate or Concentrate
- Soy Sauce or Extract

Other Sources of MSG

- MSG is found in most food prepared by major fast-food chains.
- Binders and fillers for medications, nutrients, and supplements, both prescription and non-prescription, and some fluids administered intravenously in hospitals, may contain MSG.
- According to the manufacturer, Varivax-Merck chicken pox vacinne (Varicella Virus Live) contains L-monosodium glutamate and hydrolyzed gelatin, both of which contain processed free glutamic acid.
- MSG is used as a plant "growth enhancer" (AuxiGro) that is sprayed on growing crops. AuxiGro Plant Metabolic Primer contains 29.2% by weight, pharmaceutical grade, L-glutamic acid.
- The most common sources of MSG: molasses, sugar beet & cane.
- MSG and Aspartame (NutraSweet) are found in everything from soups, sauces, and juice to frozen entrees, candy, cigarettes, and anything with seasonings (e.g., potato chips, meat, ice cream).

The following foods have enough MSG/Glutamate content to cause a reaction in individuals sensitive to it or contain some amount of Glutamate and should be avoided. Remember - ALWAYS read labels. Product contents can change at any time at the company's discretion.

Doritos
Pringles
KFC fried chicken
Boar's Head cold cuts/hot dogs
Progresso Soups
Lipton Soups/Sauces
Gravy Master
Planter's salted peanuts
Sausages/Processed meats/Cold cuts
Processed cheese spread
Molasses
Supermarket turkey & chicken (injected)
Restaurant gravy from food service cans
Ramen noodles
Boullion (any kind)
Instant soup mixes/Stocks
Many salad dressings/Croutons
Most salty, powdered dry food mixes
Flavored potato chips
Restaurant soups made from food service soup base
Gelatin
Soy sauce
Worcestershire sauce
Kombu extract
Dry milk or whey powder
Dough conditioners
Body builder protein mixes
Parmesan cheese
Fresh produce sprayed with Auxigro in the field
Some spices

Skim, 1%, 2%, non-fat, or dry milk
Whipped cream topping substitutes
Non-dairy creamers
Chocolates/Candy bars
Low-fat/Diet Foods
Cereals
Baked goods from bakeries
Frostings and fillings
Catsup
Mayonnaise
Chili sauce
Mustards
Pickles
Bottled spaghetti sauce
Citric acid (when processed from corn)
Canned and smoked tuna, oysters, clams
Barbeque sauce
Canned, frozen, or dry entrees and potpies
Fresh and frozen pizza
Flavored teas, sodas
Seasoned anything
Some peanut butters
Some bagged salads and vegetables
Tomato sauce/Stewed tomatoes
Egg substitutes
Flour
Canned refried beans
Tofu and other fermented soy products
Table salts
Anything with corn syrup added
Anything with milk solids
Anything fermented
Anything vitamin enriched
Anything protein fortified
Anything enzyme modified
Anything ultra-pasteurized

Caramel flavoring/coloring
Pectin
Cornstarch
Flowing agents
Xanthan gum/other “gums”
L-cysteine

Excitotoxin Free Diet

It is virtually impossible to completely eliminate glutamate and aspartate from your diet, nor would you want to. Stimulatory activity from the glutamate receptor is important for neurotransmission. What we want to avoid is excessive stimulation of this neurotransmitter. One way to think about excitotoxins is to imagine an empty glass Pyrex measuring cup. Understand that the cup gets filled up over the course of a day or a lifetime with glutamate. The point at which the cup is overflowing represents when you are already seeing obvious signs of neurological damage. The less that you put into the cup each day, the less likely it is to overflow. The goal of this section is to give you a good sense of the sources of glutamate and aspartate so that you can make informed choices in terms of “filling your cup”. It would be extremely difficult to follow a completely excitotoxin free diet “to the letter”. The information presented here can be used to serve as a guideline for trying to limit the intake of excitotoxins in addition to following a gluten free/casein free diet. The idea is to keep excitotoxins to a minimum; you will never avoid them completely. ***Useful resources for a decreased glutamate diet*** include Battling the MSG Myth Cookbook by Debbie Anglesey www.msgmyth.com and the PKU diet from the University of Washington http://deptswashington.edu/pku/diet.html.

High Protein Diets

All proteins contain glutamate, aspartate, and cysteine (and phenylalanine), so it is best to eat a low/moderate amount of protein, rather than a high protein diet. If you have been advised to follow the PKU (phenylalanine free) Diet, avoid or severely limit all protein-rich foods. PKU diets are designed to eliminate phenylalanine, which is a phenolic amino acid; it would be useful for phenol sensitive individuals to limit intake of phenylalanine.

Frequently, people who display Autistic type behaviors are placed on high protein diets. Because high levels of glutamate and aspartate are found naturally in protein rich foods, and excess amounts can create a wide range of bodily damage, high protein diets are not recommended for this population. The breakdown of protein also generates ammonia. Many autistic children already have issues with elevated ammonia. This is another reason to avoid high protein diets in this population.

In addition to neurological damage due to excitotoxins, high protein diets force the body into a state of cannibalism, called *Metabolic acidosis*, where blood levels become so acidic that the body starts feeding on muscle tissue for nutrients.

Vitamin K

Because Vitamin K is enzymatically involved with glutamate and sugar metabolism, it is important for people with autistic type behavior to consume foods high in this vitamin. Below is a list of Vitamin K rich foods:

Broccoli	200 mcg	Soybean oil	26.2 mcg
Spinach	106 mcg	Snap beans	24.6 mcg
Avocado	80.4 mcg	Canola oil	19.7 mcg
Turnip greens	66.8 mcg	Kiwi fruit	19.0 mcg
Lettuce	55.9 mcg	Plums	18.8 mcg
Cabbage	48.3 mcg	Green peas	17.5 mcg
Pistachio nuts	42.6 mcg	Miso	14.4 mcg
Watercress	40.4 mcg	Carrots	13.3 mcg

Sweet peppers	8.08 mcg	Celery	6.84 mcg
Potatoes	8.10 mcg	Olive oil	6.62 mcg
Tomatoes	7.38 mcg	Cauliflower	5.89 mcg
Peanut butter	7.20 mcg	Cucumbers	5.72 mcg

Sulfur

Sulfur is necessary for the metabolism of sulfur-related proteins in the body. If sulfur is deficient, an excess of nitric oxide can result, leading to excitotoxin damage. Excess sulfur can be a problem for those with CBS and SUOX mutations. Foods high in sulfur are listed below:

Red hot peppers
Fish
Meat
Legumes
Nuts
Eggs
Cabbage
Mustard leaves
Mustard/radish flowers
Dried beans
Onions
Garlic
Watercress
Horseradish
Radish
Arugula
Brussel sprouts

Molybdenum helps the body to process sulfur properly. If molybdenum levels are too low, then supplementation should be considered.

Dr. Amy's Suggestions to Support a Healthy Gut

The use of Vitamin C and Biotene toothpaste or mouthwash (available at your local pharmacy) may be useful in combating chronic streptococcal infection. The Biotene toothpaste, mouthwash and gum may also aid the mitochondria in detoxification and help to support SOD and glutathione mutations. Many individuals have issues with chronic streptococcal infection or chronic issues with other bacterial infections in the body. In addition chronic gut issues can indicate an underlying bacterial infection in the body.

Streptococcal infection in the gut can serve as a reservoir to re-infect the sinuses. Chronic streptococcal infection has been associated with OCD behavior as well as tics, over stimulatory behavior and perseverative speech. Streptococcal infection can also lay the groundwork for leaky gut which can relate to decreased weight gain or slower growth. Xylitol nasal spray will help to eliminate nasal strep, reduce ear infections and has been reported to help with leaky gut, most likely by deceasing the flow of streptococci from the sinuses into the gut. Xylitol is also available as a sugar for cooking and in Biotene gum, toothpaste and mouthwash. Another tip is to add in papaya enzyme with increased doses of Vitamin C. This helps to support the body to eliminate chronic sinus issues as well as the reservoir of strep in the gut. I suggest that you use as much papaya enzyme and Vitamin C as your body can tolerate without causing loose stools. ImmunFactor 5 once every other day will aid the body in addressing the bacterial issues as well as the use of Microbial Support RNA on a daily basis. The supplement IP6 may help to reduce stimulatory behaviors and OCD behaviors associated with chronic streptococcal infection as will the use of benfotiamine. The use of lactoferrin is also excellent to support the body in addressing streptococcal and other bacterial issues as it helps to limit the availability of iron for the microbes. This may also be helpful in reducing elevated levels of RBCs and high hematocrit values. Many microbes require the presence of iron for growth and/or virulence.

Aside from the toxic effects of mercury on the body, aluminum and lead toxicity can cause toxicity in the body. Bacteria seem to be able to hold onto aluminum. Aluminum is known to inhibit glutamate dehydrogenase which is an enzyme that converts glutamate to alpha keto glutarate. In addition aluminum interferes with the production of BH4. Therefore the presence of aluminum may be affecting levels of serotonin as well as dopamine in the body and may be affecting BH4 levels regardless of whether there is an MTHFR A1298C mutation. Malic acid, EDTA and horsetail grass are all helpful in binding aluminum in the body. As chronic bacterial infection is addressed it should help to aid in aluminum excretion.

As already mentioned, the gut may be a source or reservoir for chronic bacterial infection if it is an issue in the body. There are a number of herbs that are useful in supporting the body to address bacterial imbalances in the gut. One natural mixture that appears to work includes neem, myrrh, golden seal, cranberry, Oregon grape, barberry, uva ursi; using 1/2 to one whole capsule of each three times per day for one month (or more if needed). If a CDSA test indicates that organisms are resistant to any of these natural herbs a substitution can be made such that the resistant herbs in question can be replaced in the mixture with caprylic acid, oregamax, olive extract or GSE (grapefruit seed extract). Using a mixture of herbs such as these seven or more herbs simultaneously is less likely to lead to resistance than using single herbs to support the body in addressing microbial issues. Using seven different herbs at a time gives you the flexibility of using a small dose of each of the seven daily, or as one parent has suggested, using a different herb each day of the week at a slightly higher dose (one full capsule three times per day).

Cranberry is also excellent for support for the body to address E.coli and neem is supportive for parasites as well as for bacterial issues. Low levels of BH4 as a result of high aluminum in the body or as a result of mutations (MTHFR A1298C or CBS up regulations) can lead to more severe parasitic infections. The use of Paradex is also helpful for supporting the body to address parasites.

Rosemary, sage, juniper berry and garlic also have antimicrobial activity. While garlic is particularly useful against a range of microbes, it is a sulfur containing herb that can be a problem in high doses for those who are CBS + or SUOX – *(+/- designations relate to the nutrigenomic status as compared to the reference range used on the Genetic Profiling Systems Test Panel. +/- is a relative term*).

It is also important to support normal flora. One successful strategy is to rotate the normal flora to get a good mixture and variety. Preferred sources of normal flora include suprema dophilus, Prescript assist, kyodophilus, Ultra dairy support (even if you are not eating dairy this is a good source of flora), a sprinkle of Toueff, Colon Health Support and allerdophilus. If possible use 1/2 to 1 whole capsule of a different source of normal flora each day of the week. You can also use the Mycology Support RNA and Candex and IMF #7 once a day, as well as the Bowel Support and Stomach pH RNA to help to balance the gut. By following this plan, you create an environment where the normal flora can thrive and as a result you will help to eliminate the offending organisms. At the end of a month it is a wise idea to run a complete diagnostic stool analysis (CDSA) to confirm that the gut flora is in balance.

In addition to its role in pancreatic support, CCK also appears to aid in addressing chronic bacterial loads in the body. As a result, the dose that is tolerated will depend in part on the bacterial load in your system. In order to use the CCK to address chronic bacterial issues it may require a much higher dose than the 1/4 tablet used only for pancreatic support. I suggest that you consider increasing the dose slowly from the 1/4 per day. You will get a sense over time of the maximum dose needed to help to aid in chronic bacterial issues. I suggest you consider starting with the 1/4 tablet along with 1/6 dropper CCK Support and gradually increase the CCK tablet by 1/4 amounts over time to three per day.

It is important if you have a history of problems keeping the gut flora in balance, to look at implementing all three aspects of the gut program.

- The use of Bowel support, Stomach pH, CCK/BioThyro (or alternating BioThyro with low dose prescription BH4), and malic acid/EDTA/horsetail grass is also designed to help change the gut environment so it is less conducive to the growth of non-ideal organisms and encourages the long-term growth of beneficial organisms. That combination should also help to chelate aluminum that is excreted as a function of elimination of imbalanced/dysbiotic flora.

- The use of a mixture of normal flora is designed to help to colonize the gut with a variety of normal flora. I have found that using the concept of rotating the sources of normal flora helps in establishing a nice balance of gut flora.

- The third arm of the gut program is to help to eliminate non-ideal gut microbes. The use of the mixture of gut herbs (tailored to reflect the sensitivity testing results seen on a CDSA), along with the microbial support formula, IMF 5 and lactoferrin is designed to address bacterial imbalances. In a similar fashion the use of the mycology support formula, along with Candex, herbs as noted on a CDSA sensitivity test, IMF 7, and lactoferrin is designed to address yeast imbalances.

The situation regarding the bacterium Clostridium deserves special mention. There is some indication that Clostridia infection may have an impact on language. A severe expressive language delay was noted for an autistic child with a duplication of 28 genes on chromosome 7 (NEJM. 353:1694, 2005). This is the identical region that is deleted in children with Williams Beuren Syndrome, a condition that is characterized by accelerated language development. The implication is that one of these 28 genes plays a role in language. As I discussed at the conference in February, 2006 in Arizona, a close inspection of these 28 genes yields several candidates that may be involved in the apraxia noted in the autistic child with the gene duplication. Two of the 28 genes are involved in the binding of Clostridia toxins. In addition, I have come across a recent case where very high Clostridia levels were associated with decreased language for an individual. This does suggest that high levels of this anaerobic bacterium may play a role in limited language. There are several types of tests available to ascertain if Clostridia infection in the gut is an issue. Particular OAT/MAT tests indicate the levels of HPHPA, which is described to be elevated with Clostridia infection. Levels of DHPPA on other OAT/MAT tests have formerly been discussed as relating to Clostridia levels. Since there continues to be some disagreement over the implication of the levels of these biochemical intermediates and their relationship to Clostridia levels, it is wise to run a specific stool test to confirm the presence of Clostridia toxins if you see elevated levels of HPHPA or DHPPA listed on an OAT/MAT test. Clostridium is an anaerobe, which means that it does not grow well (if at all) in a high oxygen environment. Approaches for addressing Clostridia in the gut include the use of Oxydrene (1/2 once or twice daily), O2 Plus, Cell food (2 to 3 drops daily), Penta water; the herb bay leaf has been reported to be very effective against Clostridia, and Florastor to replace the presence of Clostridia with normal flora. An apraxia support formula is also under development at this time. Addressing Clostridia infection may also help with loose stools. The toxins excreted by Clostridia cause gaps between the cells lining the gut, adding to leaky gut issues.

Loose stools are an issue for a number of individuals, and I do understand that the SCD (Specific Carbohydrate Diet) has made a big difference in these cases. However, if you are supplementing protein it is important to monitor ammonia levels to be certain that the body is able to dispose of the ammonia properly that is generated from the intake of high protein foods. The body uses two molecules of BH4 to detoxify one molecule of ammonia to urea. This is an "expensive" way to use your BH4. BH4 is also needed for dopamine and serotonin synthesis, as well as language related function. Adequate levels of GABA, BH4, and dopamine appear to play a major role in language development. Since language is a primary problem for many children, using up limited BH4 to detoxify ammonia may not be the best use of it for the body. In addition, ammonia is reported to inhibit the metabolism of butyrate, along with other short chain fatty acids. Butyrate is a nutrient used by cells that line the gut. Butyrate synthesis can be inhibited by H2S and sulfites that are generated as a result of the CBS up regulation, low molybdenum or SUOX mutations. Paradoxically, butyrate has been reported to be a potent detoxifier of ammonia. Excess ammonia can also deplete manganese stores in the body as manganese is needed to help to detoxify ammonia. Classic signs of chronic manganese deficiency include low cholesterol, elevated alkaline phosphatase levels and depressed T-cell mediated immune function (due to thymus issues). In addition, manganese is needed to produce dopamine as well as for Vitamin C to function in the body. The pancreas requires manganese for insulin production. A lack of acetylcholine and difficulty entering the Krebs cycle is related to low levels of manganese. It is particularly important to monitor manganese levels as well as molybdenum levels for individuals with CBS mutations.

Excess stomach acid in the system can cause loose stools and severe stomach pain. Ammonia that is generated from excessive protein is alkaline. This may help to neutralize the stomach acid and would make the stools and gut pain better. However, using a high protein diet to address loose stools is not dealing with the root of the problem if it is caused by excess stomach acid. Creating high ammonia levels via diet to neutralize acids treats the symptom but not the underlying imbalance in the body. Stomach acid is triggered by histamine reacting with H2 receptors in the stomach. So a high protein diet may be increasing ammonia which is neutralizing the stomach acid and improving the gut issue. However, it is not addressing why you have excess acid in the first place nor is it considering why there may be high histamine in the system (histamine is related to methylation function). In addition it is important to evaluate ammonia levels and to consider the consequences of high ammonia. I am not suggesting that individuals abandon the SCD diet, especially as it has made a positive difference for many people. However, I would suggest a test for Helicobacter pylori as that is often a causative agent for excess stomach acid (stool tests are now available in addition to the saliva test). The use of mastica gum is reported to be very helpful for addressing this organism. I would suggest ½ mastica gum, Stomach pH and Bowel support with meals. I would also suggest that you consider running a DDI urine amino acid test so that you can look at ammonia levels and amino acids while on the SCD diet.

Acid reflux seen in individuals with SUOX mutations or with CBS up regulations may be related to the excess sulfites in their systems. Maintaining adequate levels of molybdenum, limiting sulfur donors, and the use of the lung support formula, respiratory support formula as well as the stomach pH formula, stress and hyperimmune formulas may be beneficial in helping to balance the acid reflux. The use of urine test strips to monitor sulfite and sulfate levels is also helpful. (Using test strips to measure copper levels is another indirect indication of molybdenum depletion. Additional test strips are available for iron and nickel levels. These test strips are not meant to replace the need for urine toxic and essential mineral screening, rather as more immediate feedback mechanisms between urine samples). Quercetin can be used to limit mast cell degranulation for those individuals who are COMT - - or COMT + -. In addition, Petadulex (butterbur) may be helpful in balancing allergic/histamine reactions. Several of the individuals that have presented with a SUOX + - status have also complained of severe acid reflux that seems to be non responsive (or showing only limited responsiveness) to more classic medications for Gastroesophageal reflux (GER). Standard medications for acid reflux tend to be targeted at the mechanism that triggers excess acid in the stomach (histamine 2 blockers). It is possible that for individuals with SUOX issues, that the root of the problem is the excess sulfites creating allergic/asthmatic type reactions that have a secondary effect on acid reflux. Gastroesophageal reflux (GER) occurs commonly in patients with asthma and a relationship between asthma and acid reflux had been noted for quite some time. It is uncertain whether the asthma causes the acid reflux, or if the converse is true. High sulfites are known triggers for asthma. There are some indications that the sequence of events that occur in asthma may lead to the excess acid production. Ordinarily, we think of histamine reactions as allergic reactions; however, it is important to realize that it is over activity by histamine receptors that is tied to the excess acid production observed in GERD. According to Pneumological Aspects of Gastroesophageal Reflux (edited by Dal Negro and Allegra). "*Gastroesophageal reflux (GER) refers to symptoms and events that result from abnormal regurgitation of gastric contents into the esophagus. Respiratory diseases, in particular bronchial asthma, can be exacerbated by multiple triggers, including GER. The relationship between the occurrence of gastroesophageal disorders and changes in respiratory function has been known for over a century, but the mechanism by which esophageal acid regurgitation can produce respiratory symptoms is still debated. The reasons for these concurrent pathological events are also not fully understood. Determining, for instance, whether reflux itself initiates or exacerbates asthma, or whether asthma or its treatment primarily causes GER is a matter of current investigation.*"

The potential effect of excess sulfites on acid reflux is not to minimize the effect that heavy metal toxicity and chronic viral infection can have on potential acid reflux. Acid reflux may also tie in directly with chronic viral infection in the body. Cimetidine (Tagament), an OTC medication for heartburn, has been demonstrated to have efficacy against herpes virus (LEF March 2001). This would suggest that chronic viral infection may also play a role in acid reflux. The use of OTC heartburn medication may appear to aggravate the condition, while in actuality it may be acting to aid in viral detoxification and the concomitant release of metals from the system. The use of urine toxic metals tests are useful in determining if this is indeed the case.

On a related note other helpful tools for addressing bacterial and viral infection and supporting the body in the process include the use of Ora Triplex, Immuno Forte, Moducare and the ImmunFactors (IMF). In particular IMF 4 should be helpful for viruses related to childhood vaccines. The IMF 1, 2 and 6 should be helpful in supporting the body for herpes related viruses and I have found that the IMF 5 works nicely for support of bacterial infections.

Those individuals with CBS up regulations should limit their use of IMFs to one per day due to lipid acting components in the product.

Chronic bacterial infection and its effects on tryptophan breakdown are part of the reason why I suggest only low levels of P5P for individuals with chronic bacterial issues and CBS up regulations. P5P also helps to push the CBS reaction as well as to aid in the conversion of kynurenic to quinolinic. The kynurenic that is generated via the breakdown of tryptophan by bacterial infection is calming; however P5P helps to convert it to quinolinic which is excitatory.

In animal models, Vitamin B2 (riboflavin) has been shown to speed the clearance of bacteria from the body and to lower mortality rates from bacterial sepsis. In addition, riboflavin is reported to be helpful in reducing inflammatory mediators. Another B vitamin, Vitamin B3, is often depleted in individuals with chronic bacterial infections. You may also want to consider niacinamide (1/2 per day) as this may help to stem the breakdown of tryptophan that is often seen with bacterial infection. Kynurenate is part of the breakdown pathway for tryptophan. As the body breaks down tryptophan for this purpose it will also deplete serotonin. Lack of serotonin combined with streptococcal infection can lead to perseverative and OCD behaviors in addition to other effects. The mao A gene, codes for the enzyme involved in serotonin breakdown. Individuals with a mao A + status may show decreased enzyme activity such that mao A is less effective in degrading serotonin. This may mean that OCD type behaviors may be less of a problem or less noticeable, even if chronic bacterial infection is an issue. This may also be reflected in higher levels of serotonin, tryptophan or lower levels of 5 hydroxy indole acetic acid (5HIAA) on organic acid tests and urine amino acid tests. The final breakdown product of the tryptophan pathway is niacinamide. This B vitamin has been reported to have antimicrobial effects. It may be that the body is trying to address bacterial infection by breaking down tryptophan into niacinamide to help with infection. In some cases I have not found that the use of high dose B6 or P5P is always helpful. It can actually cause more overstimulatory or OCD type behaviors. While kynurenic acid is calming for neuro-transmitters, the product that kynurenines are converted to by B6 is quinolinic acid. Quinolinic acid is an excitotoxin. So, if you have high kynurenine and add B6 you can generate quinolinic acid which acts as an excitotoxin and can aggravate the nervous system. Increased levels of quinolinic acid have been implicated in Alzheimer's disease as well as with respect to excitotoxin damage of nerves. Quinolinic acid was found to be substantially elevated in patients with Borrelia burgdorferi (Lyme) infection and has been postulated to play a role in contributing to neurological and cognitive defects associated with Lyme disease. It is of importance to try to look at why you may have elevated activity in the tryptophan breakdown pathway in the first place. Decreased methylation, increased IDO (an enzyme that is also effected by methylation and other factors), and chronic streptococcal or even B. burgdorferi (Lyme) infection can lead to stimulation of this pathway.

A future consideration may be to look at addressing the possibility of chronic Lyme infection in the body. Lyme disease has been implicated in a number of neurological conditions. Cat's Claw is reported to be helpful for viral issues as well as for Lyme. Artemisia (wormwood) has also shown activity against Lyme. Wormwood is a component of Paradex that was already mentioned with respect to other parasitic infections. In addition, tick support RNAs and IMF 2 should help to support the body. Chronic issues with Lyme may overlap with thyroid dysfunction.

There is a complex relationship between thyroid function and bacterial infection. Healthy thyroid activity helps to address chronic bacterial/sinus infection. Conversely, the presence of chronic bacterial infection can impair thyroid hormone levels, creating a bit of a catch 22. Periodic thyroid tests and CDSAs to assess the status of bacterial infection and its effect on thyroid function are suggested for individuals who have issues with chronic bacterial infection, sinus infections, dental issues, or a past history of ear infections. One of the enzymes that is activated during chronic bacterial infection is also needed for thyroid hormone synthesis. Since low thyroid function is often found in association with a variety of neurological and cardiovascular conditions, I felt this was a good time to raise potential problems so that you can be aware of them and watch for signs of these on issues in the future. Iodine levels also affect thyroid function and there is a relationship between the methylation cycle, sulfur groups and iodine levels. Iodine levels will be impacted negatively by bromine that is used in bread. This is another reason to be vigilant with the gluten free aspect of the GF/CF diet. Lithium is concentrated in the thyroid and can inhibit iodine uptake. This is why it is important to monitor both the levels of iodine as well as lithium on essential mineral tests and supplement lithium only as needed for low values that may occur as a result of detoxification and excretion of mercury. Iodine is no longer included on the standard essential element test, and needs to be ordered as a separate test. As an alternative, a topical iodine test can be performed.

If iodine and thyroid hormone levels are an issue, the use of ½ to one Iodoral per day may be of help in supporting healthy iodine levels. The use of the herb guggul may help to balance T3 and T4. Natural thyroid supplementation is available in the form of thyroid/tyrosine supplements. After four to six weeks of nutritional support you should run a follow up thyroid test with your health care provider to confirm that thyroid hormone levels are in the normal range and an essential mineral iodine test to confirm healthy iodine levels (or the use of the topical iodine test). The thyroid hormone iodination cycle is tied to glucose 6 phosphate dehydrogenase levels. The use of supplements or chelating agents that deplete G6PDH levels can also affect thyroid hormone levels.

Chronic streptococcal infection, and possibly E.coli infection can also lead to a variety of inflammatory mediators as well as depleting neurotransmitters. Bacterial infection is also known to increase the levels of inflammatory mediators such as IL6 and TNF alpha. Mutations have been characterized that aid in increasing the levels IL6 or TNF alpha in the system. Elevated IL6 has been reported to inhibit the release of thyroid hormones in addition to its role in enhancing inflammation. The use of Health Foundation RNA, Vitamin K, Kidney Support RNA, nettle, boswellia, Behavior

Support RNAs and skullcap may help to balance the body so that these mediators are less of an issue. In addition, curcumin and green tea may be helpful (not for COMT ++ individuals).

In addition to its reported effect on IL6, Vitamin K may also be useful in supporting blood sugar imbalances. The Fok + status for the VDR (Vitamin D receptor) has been associated with potential blood sugar issues. Vitamin D levels are also closely tied to a variety of neurological conditions. Based on recent literature, individuals should consider supplementing with at least 1000 IU of supplemental Vitamin D daily. Also, the use of 1/6 dropper of Pro Longevity RNA has proven to be helpful for many individuals. Vitamin K and supplements to support the pancreas should also be considered such as OraPancreas, Gymnema sylvestre, Super Digestive enzymes, CCK (see below) and the supplement called pig duodenum. The essential minerals chromium and vanadium also play a role in blood sugar levels. It is important to watch the level of these minerals and look at adding chromium picolinate and vanadyl if their levels drop on an essential mineral test. Since low blood sugar can trigger seizure activity for those that are susceptible to it, it is wise to support the pancreas for individuals who are VDR/Fok+. In addition to effects on blood sugar, variations in the VDR Fok marker reflect differences in bone mineral density. While increased bone mineral density is associated with increased calcium absorption it has also been associated with higher blood concentrations of lead. I initially suggested the use of CCK to aid in supporting the pancreas. For mere pancreatic support it should be sufficient to use 1/4 to 1/2 CCK, the CCK Support RNA (1/8 dropper), OraPancreas (2 to 3 per day), Super Digestive enzymes and pig duodenum with meals, and gymnema sylvestre. The newest addition for pancreatic support is the use of methyl pyruvate. (To digress for a moment, the methyl pyruvate does trigger additional detox as well as supporting the pancreas. I suggest that if you choose to add methyl pyruvate to your program that you add it as a separate item as it is another variable. Follow the directions on the bottle for dilution of the methyl pyruvate and then I suggest starting with 1/4 of the suggested dose of the already diluted material.)

In addition to effects on blood sugar levels, decreased pancreatic activity may be associated with increased levels of oxalic acid as measured on organic acid tests. Supplementation to support healthy blood sugar levels and the pancreas may also be helpful in normalizing increased oxalic acid. In addition, the use of the herbs Sheep sorrel and Turkey rhubarb may contribute to elevated levels of oxalic acid

Individuals showing elevated oxalic acid along with elevated triglycerides on lab work may indicate a need for both pancreatic as well as liver support. Liver support can include OraLiv, OraTriplex, Milk Thistle and Dandelion Root.

On a related note, pantothenic acid, molybdenum and quercetin (no quercetin for COMT V158M + +) may be helpful for elevated uric acid along with supplementation to support the kidneys (Kidney Support RNA, OraKidney, dandelion leaf).

About the Authors

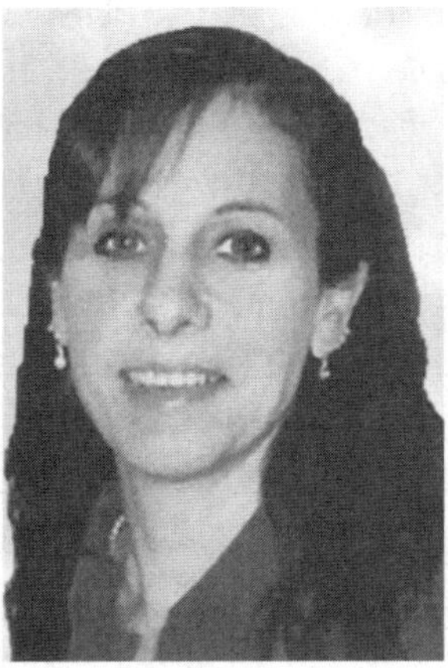

Amy A. Yasko Ph.D., ND, NHD, AMD, HHP, FAAIM, has extensive expertise in biochemistry, molecular biology, and biotechnology. She also has research and clinical experience in both allopathic and alternative medicine. The common thread that winds through these fields is her work with RNA.

As co-founder and owner of a successful biotechnology company, she is recognized as an expert in molecular biology in the field of DNA/RNA based diagnostics and therapeutics and has been a consultant to the medical and research community for eighteen years. More than twenty years ago she began isolating single copy RNA messages from transformed cells at Strong Memorial Hospital Cancer Center. Later while at Yale Medical Center she worked to enhance the expression of specific eukaryotic RNAs from yeast.

During her tenure at St. Vincent's Hospital in NYC, Dr. Yasko developed custom diets and used nutritional supplements to improve the cure rates of Hodgkin's disease patients. She worked with Dr. Lawrence to isolate some of the first clinical samples of Transfer Factor for use in these patients. She then went on to conduct molecular research on Transfer Factor in Dr. Fudenburg's Immunology Dept. at the Medical University of South Carolina.

Dr. Yasko was also a member of the Dept. of Pediatrics and Infectious Diseases at Strong Memorial Hospital and worked to develop safer *Haemophilus influenza* vaccines. She has also spent years studying the relationship between energy transport and modes of antibiotic resistance by bacteria and has written articles and chapters in books on the subject.

Dr. Yasko then established an alternative healthcare practice specializing in chronic inflammation, immunological and neurological disorders. To date she has had considerable success in halting and in most cases reversing the effects of such debilitating diseases from which her clients suffer, such as ALS, MS, Parkinson's disease, Alzheimer's disease, SLE, Myasthenia gravis and autism. Most recently her primary focus has been to construct a program to help to reverse autism.

Dr. Yasko graduated cum laude with a BS in Chemistry and Fine Arts from Colgate University. She then completed her medical education at Albany Medical College and received a Doctorate in Microbiology, Immunology and Infectious Diseases with an award for outstanding academic excellence, graduating summa cum laude. She was the first woman in that department to receive a Doctorate in this field. Dr. Yasko continued her education to graduate with high honors from the Clayton College of Natural Health, receiving two additional degrees, a Doctor of Naturopathy and a Doctor of Natural Health. She is licensed as a Naturopathic Physician and board certified as an Alternative Medical Doctor, a Holistic Health Practitioner and is a Fellow of the American Association of Integrative Medicine. She was the recipient of the 2004 CASD award for RNA Research in autism.

Dr. Yasko has coauthored the book *Heal Your Body Naturally: The Power of RNA* and is the author of *Genetic Bypass*, a book that describes the use of nutrition to bypass genetic mutations. She lives in Maine with her husband and three children.

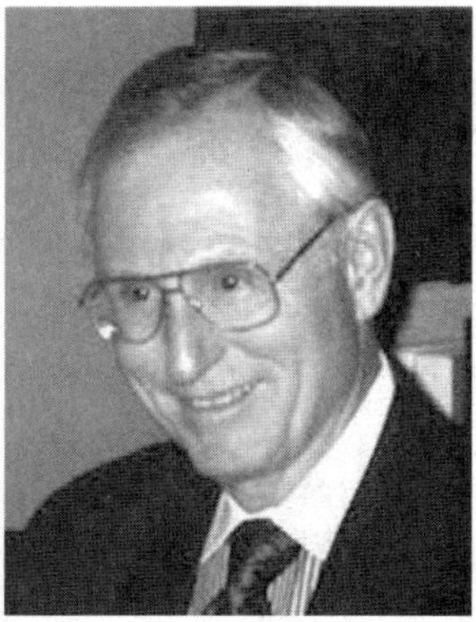

Garry F. Gordon MD, DO, MD (H), received his Doctor of Osteopathy in 1958 from the Chicago College of Osteopathy in Illinois. He received his honorary MD degree from the University of California Irvine in 1962 and completed his Radiology Residency from Mt. Zion in San Francisco, California in 1964. For many years, he was the Medical Director of Mineral Lab in Hayward, California, a leading laboratory for trace mineral analysis worldwide with offices in Boston, Amsterdam, and Tokyo.

Dr. Gordon is on the Board of Homeopathic Medical Examiners for Arizona and is Co-Founder of the American College for Advancement in Medicine (ACAM). He is Founder/President of the International College of Advanced Longevity (ICALM) and Board Member of International Oxidative Medicine Association (IOMA). He is also a member of the Scientific Advisory Committee for The National Foundation for Alternative Medicine.

With Morton Walker, DPM, Dr. Gordon co-authored *The Chelation Answer*. In addition, he was the instructor and examiner for all chelation physicians. Currently he is an advisor to the American Board of Chelation Therapy and responsible for Peer Review for Chelation Therapy in the State of Arizona.

As an internationally recognized expert on chelation therapy, Dr. Gordon is now attempting to establish standards for the proper use of oral and intravenous chelation therapy as an adjunct therapy for all diseases. He lectures extensively on *The End Of Bypass Surgery Is In Sight* and *The Future of Chelation.*

Currently, Dr. Gordon is President of Gordon Research Institute and a full-time consultant for Longevity Plus, a nutritional supplement company located in Payson, Arizona. He is responsible for the design of the majority of their supplements, which are widely used by alternative health practitioners around the world.